Being An Empowered Patient

An Advocacy Guide

Medical Malpractice, Technology and Other Essential Topics

Erika Balfour MD

Being An Empowered Patient
An Advocacy Guide
Medical Malpractice, Technology and Other Essential Topics

Dedication

For family, friends and country

Contents

Preface

THIS BOOK IS WRITTEN FOR THE benefit of the patient and is therefore entitled "Being An Empowered Patient: An Advocacy Guide". The mission of this book is to successfully direct its readers through the mysteries and frustrations surrounding healthcare. I hope to not only shed light on the complexities of this experience, but to provide the reader with useful tools to get the best medical outcome. Ultimately, the reader should no longer have despair with regards to healthcare, but in fact should be stronger, wiser and therefore more satisfied with their medical experience.

I encourage you to take charge and empower yourself with regards to your health. Start by becoming a team player; join the medical team treating you. You can accomplish this by knowing basics about healthcare, your condition, insurance companies and the legal system. This may seem like a daunting task, but after reading this book, you will be well versed in all mentioned. Your doctor will be inspired by your enthusiasm and initiative and will welcome you to the team.

This book can be read from cover to cover, or alternatively, as a reference book. The latter allows you to choose to read the chapter most relevant at that time in your life. Each chapter offers insight for you to maximize your healthcare experience.

Introduction

WELCOME TO AN INSIDE LOOK INTO the world of medicine. Written by a medical doctor, this book offers explanations to confusing medical language and situations. Solutions and tips are given so that the patient is ultimately more equipped to address medical concerns. Methods are explored to smoothly navigate through the patient's medical journey. This book includes a 'real' assessment of healthcare that does not blindly support medical professionals, agencies or policies. This unique and comprehensive perspective includes:

Chapter 1.
Basic Medical Knowledge
There are basic concepts that are critical for a patient to grasp in order to maximize his/her healthcare experience. Such concepts include differentiating between; a symptom and a diagnosis; a primary care doctor and a specialist; doctors and other healthcare professionals; traditional medicine and alternative medicine.

Chapter 2.
Doctor Selection

This unique chapter offers the patient an opportunity to learn the difference between healthcare professionals and consequently, make better choices for his/her condition. This chapter also explains that there are doctors who participate in the patient's care, unbeknownst to the patient.

Chapter 3.
Preparation For The First Medical Visit

The importance of building a positive relationship with a patient's doctor is exemplified in this chapter along with tips on how to accomplish this task. Solutions to potential barriers of care, such as language, transportation and cultural differences are also reviewed.

Chapter 4.
During The Medical Visit

Emphasis is placed on patient honesty and ensuring that the healthcare professional has recorded accurate information in the patient's medical note and chart.

Chapter 5.
After The Medical Visit

There are many decisions a patient must make after seeing a doctor. For example, a patient must decide if he/she will follow the doctor's orders or choose to end the relationship and seek other professional advice. Additionally, a patient may seek the help of family and friends to get the medical and social support they are in need of. A patient's understanding of his/her own condition can relieve some anxiety.

Chapter 6.
Medical Insurance: What To Know

Given the complexities surrounding medical insurance in our nation, this chapter attempts to simplify it and focuses on key points necessary to make more informed choices.

Chapter 7.
Disability Insurance: What To Know

This chapter demonstrates the need for disability insurance and provides information regarding claim denial and reversal.

Chapter 8.
Medical Fraud And Medical Malpractice

Legal criteria for medical fraud and medical malpractice are presented. There is a discussion of what action a patient can undertake if he/she suspects medical fraud or malpractice.

Chapter 9.
Trends In Healthcare

This chapter highlights developing concepts in healthcare including electronic medical records, the use of social media, and new potential technologies for therapy- such as stem cells, targeted molecular medicine, gene therapy and 3D printing for organ transplants.

1

Basic Medical Knowledge

IN ORDER TO GET THE MOST out of your healthcare experience, you should have basic medical knowledge. Obtaining knowledge about the concepts addressed in this chapter will provide you with a strong foundation for all future medical encounters.

1.1 Symptom vs. Diagnosis

Many patients do not know the difference between a symptom and a diagnosis. This section is designed to explain the difference and the importance of this distinction.

"My stomach hurts"
" I have the worst headache"
" Pain is radiating down my leg"
" The whites of my eyes are yellow"

These descriptions are what medical professionals call *symptoms*. Symptoms are the reflection of what is going awry with the body. By analyzing your symptom(s), the doctor is able to narrow down the possible causes of your problem and eventually determine the one cause. The one cause is called the *diagnosis*. Therefore, a symptom is not a diagnosis but is rather a description. A symptom describes the diagnosis. The diagnosis is the actual cause of the disease, while the symptom is the effect.

1.1.1 Symptoms Identify the Diagnosis

A doctor is like a detective; he/she can only solve the mystery after analyzing all of the clues and putting the pieces together. For a doctor, the clues are represented by symptoms. By putting all of the clues or symptoms together, the doctor can solve the mystery, that is, determine the diagnosis. Thus, many diagnoses require the analysis of multiple symptoms before a single diagnosis can be reached.

In some cases, additional tests, namely laboratory (blood work, biopsy) and radiographic tests (x-rays, MRI, CAT scans) may be required to determine the diagnosis.

1.1.2 Diagnosis Without a Symptom

Usually, the diagnosis is made after you relay your symptom(s) to your doctor. But in some circumstances, the doctor may inform you of a diagnosis after performing a routine examination, without any symptom. For example, during a routine medical visit, your doctor found a skin cancer behind your ear. You had not previously seen it. In this case, the skin cancer was diagnosed without symptoms.

1.1.3 Are You Being Treated for Your Symptom or Diagnosis?

In general, once the diagnosis has been made, a doctor treats you based on your diagnosis (cause of the disease), not the symptoms. However, if there is no cure or if the cure is not possible at that time, then the doctor will treat the symptoms (effect of the disease). Treating the symptoms is often not meant to cure you but may make you feel better, if only temporarily. Treatment of symptoms therefore is often meant to resolve secondary problems that were caused by a diagnosis. Treatment of a diagnosis, on the other hand, is generally meant to cure. Some patients may not realize that only their symptoms are being treated, which means the actual cause of their problem remains and in some cases may worsen over time without direct treatment. This demonstrates the importance for you to know the difference between your symptoms and your diagnosis. You should ask your doctor directly, "What is my diagnosis?" If you are unsure as to whether the response represents a diagnosis or a symptom, the next question to the doctor should be: "That is my diagnosis, not my symptom, correct?". Example 1, in this chapter, clarifies this concept.

Example 1. Basic Medical Knowledge: Are You Being Treated for Your Symptom or Diagnosis?
<u>Scenario:</u> A 62-year-old man had pain and tightness in his lower back that radiated down his left leg. A MRI was performed and showed a spinal disc herniation (slipped disc) in his lower back. In this scenario, the following are true:

Symptom: lower back pain
Diagnosis: slipped disc
Treatment of symptom: physical therapy, medication
  (muscle relaxants, anti-inflammatory), and/or
  medical injections
Treatment of diagnosis: neurosurgical procedure
  (disc fusion, etc.)

<u>Discussion:</u> The options listed above for treating the symptoms can be long term, with the symptoms recurring and sometimes worsening over time. The option for treating the diagnosis, on the other hand, if successful, may cure the problem.

This example demonstrates the difference between a symptom and a diagnosis. It also shows how some treatment options target symptoms, while others target the diagnosis.

(Note: This example does not take into consideration the severity of the disc herniation, if surgery would be an appropriate option, or the side effects of treating the symptom and possible complications from surgery.)

> **KEY POINT:** The decision to treat the symptom versus the diagnosis is based on all of the cumulative health information that your doctor analyzes for your particular case. Ensure that you understand which is being treated, your symptom or diagnosis.

1.2   Who are Primary Care Doctors?

Choosing the right doctor to treat your condition is very important. Many patients do not know the difference between primary care doctors and specialists. Some patients have found out the hard way, that is, saw a specialist without a referral from a primary care doctor, and were then responsible for a hefty bill, as some Health Management Organizations (HMOs) and government insurance policies do not cover specialist visits without a referral [1].

Primary care is the medical attention provided to you that does not require specialized medical intervention. Primary care doctors complete three or four years of training after medical school. These doctors are then eligible for board certification by their respective national board organization.

Primary care doctors provide the foundation needed to treat common conditions. Conditions such as colds, ear infections, hypertension, diabetes, and uncomplicated broken bones are examples of routine medical cases. These conditions have a somewhat standard protocol for treatment. Yet, even these conditions may present themselves as, or later become, complicated. In such cases, the primary care doctor may refer the patient to a specialist.

The various types of primary care doctors differentiate themselves by the number of years trained and the patient populations served. Of course, an older doctor practicing for many years should have more "hands-on" experience treating patients than a doctor that has recently graduated from medical school.

Please see Table A, Type of Primary Care Doctors, for a limited list of primary care doctors and some of the diseases/conditions they treat.

Table A.
Type of Primary Care Doctors (abridged list)

Doctor	Treatment (of) And Patient Age
Family Practitioner	Common conditions (Any age)
Internist	Common conditions (18 yrs. old to death)
Pediatrician	Common conditions that afflict children and young adults (Birth to 18-21 yrs.)
Obstetrician/ Gynecologist	Pregnant female patients, child birth, genetics, sexually transmitted infections, cancer screening of female organs (21 yrs. of age to death, sometimes teens)
Geriatrician	Conditions that afflict the elderly while addressing malnutrition, mental senility, disabilities, multiple-drug therapies (65 yrs. old or older)

Reviewing Table A shows that **DIFFERENT** types of primary care doctors can treat the **SAME** diseases. This begs the question: how do you choose which type of primary care doctor to see? The answer is based on which patient population the doctor studied during training and the overall length of time the doctor trained. Example 2, in this chapter, addresses this concept.

Example 2. Basic Medical Knowledge: Who are Primary Care Doctors?

Scenario: A 29-year-old woman had a chronic cough. Should she seek help from a family practitioner or an internist?

Discussion: Both types of doctors are qualified to address this issue. If the patient does not have an option, either type of physician would be fine. However, if a patient has an option, one choice may be better than the other. This decision is dependent on such factors as the age of the patient. For example, if the patient is ten years old, perhaps a family practitioner would be recommended. If, on the other hand, the patient is a middle-aged chronic smoker who has been in and out of the hospital due to other health issues, perhaps the patient should be seen by an internist. Although a family practitioner is well qualified to treat the patient in this scenario, because an internist specializes in the treatment of adult diseases, this patient may want to opt for the internist.

1.2.1 How to Distinguish Between Various Primary Care Doctors

There are differences between the various types of primary care doctors. These differences are based on which field the doctor trained in. You should recognize these differences so that you can choose a doctor that is best qualified to address your medical concerns. Below are brief descriptions of the training each type of doctor has undertaken. You can use these descriptions as a reference before making your next primary care doctor appointment. (Example 3, in this chapter, exemplifies the thought process when choosing a primary care doctor.)

Family Medicine or Internal Medicine?

A family medicine doctor, otherwise known as a family practitioner, trains in family medicine. This includes, but is not limited to, surgery, pediatrics, geriatrics, ob-gyn (obstetrics and gynecology), and medical clinics. Alternatively, an internal medicine doctor, otherwise known as an internist, trains in the same disciplines but focuses on the treatment of adult diseases. A family practice doctor usually practices in an office/clinic setting and rarely in a hospital while an internist can be found in an office/clinic setting and often in a hospital.

Family medicine doctors can further enhance their training by obtaining additional certification in various disciplines such as sleep medicine, sports medicine, geriatrics, and adolescent medicine. Internal medicine doctors, on the other hand, can subspecialize (get more training), in disciplines like cardiology, gastroenterology, neurology, endocrinology, etc. These subspecialties concentrate on internal conditions, or organ systems.

Family Medicine or Pediatrics?
If you are younger than 21 years old, a pediatrician may be preferred given the years of focused training in this population. However, a family medicine doctor is qualified to treat patients in this age group as well.

Family Medicine or Obstetrician/Gynecology (OB-GYN)?
If you seek advice/treatment regarding female reproductive organs, an obstetrician/gynecologist may be preferred given the years of focused training in this population. However, a family medicine doctor is qualified to treat patients in this age group as well. However, if your pregnancy is not routine (high risk), for example, you are older when pregnant, have a chronic condition, such as diabetes or hypertension, or develop complications while pregnant, an obstetrician/gynecologist is highly recommended. In such cases, the family medicine doctor may refer you to an obstetrician/gynecologist. (For some insurance policies, obstetrician/gynecology is not considered primary care and falls under specialist care.)

Example 3. Basic Medical Knowledge: Who are Primary Care Doctors?

Scenario: A 13–year-old girl started her period. As her parent, you must decide if she should be seen by a family practitioner/general practitioner, pediatrician or OB/GYN (obstetrician/gynecologist)?

Discussion: All three types of doctors are equipped with the knowledge to treat this patient. You can choose which doctor would be best based on the other factors, such as your daughter's comfort level. Perhaps the young patient would like to continue seeing her family doctor or pediatrician, since she has known this doctor for some time. Alternatively, the young patient may see this as an opportunity to visit an OB/GYN (obstetrician/gynecologist) for privacy, away from her family. The point is that all three types of doctors are fully able to successfully treat this patient and that you can choose best by examining what your daughter needs in order to feel the most comfortable.

Family Medicine/Internal Medicine or Geriatrics?

If you are over the age of 65, a geriatrician may be preferred. This is because a geriatrician has spent 1-2 years studying and treating patients that are 65 and older. However, a family medicine/internist doctor is qualified to treat patients in this age group as well. Keep in mind that there are many patients that are considered "young old" (over the age of 65 and have no serious or unstable disabling disease) [2]. These people may choose not to be seen by a geriatrician and are relatively healthy as they maintain proper nutrition, exercise and mental status. Also, older patients may feel more comfortable continuing their care with a family medicine/internist doctor they have known for many years.

1.3 Who are Medical Specialists?

Specialized medicine is the medical attention provided to you that requires more than basic medical intervention. It builds on the foundation that is practiced by primary care doctors. It is care offered to you that requires treatment from an expert doctor that has trained to treat particular diseases/conditions.

A specialist, therefore, can perform highly skilled tests, procedures and/or surgery, order and interpret sophisticated laboratory tests and treat both rare and complicated conditions. A primary care doctor can refer you to a specialist, however, some medical insurance policies permit you to see a specialist without first consulting a primary care doctor. Be sure to check the stipulations regarding this with your own medical insurance policy.

Like primary care doctors, the various types of specialists differentiate themselves by the patient populations served and the number of years trained. All specialists complete three or four years of training after medical school. These doctors are then eligible for board certification by their respective national board organization. (Please keep in mind that primary care doctors may also be specialists if they have taken additional training in a particular specialty. This is exemplified in the Internal Medicine Specialties list within Table B. Type of Medical Specialists.)

Finally, if you or your doctor decide that you require a specialist for your condition, be sure to understand why and what that specialist can offer you. The type of illness dictates what type of specialist is needed. Table B, Type of Medical Specialists lists some specialists and the services they provide.

Table B.
Type of Medical Specialists (abridged list)

Medical Specialists (Type)	Treatment (of)
Colon and Rectal Surgeon	Removal of colon and rectal cancer, hemorrhoids
Dermatologist	Skin, nail and hair disorders
Emergency Medicine	Urgent healthcare
General Surgeon	Appendicitis, gallbladder removal
Internal Medicine Specialties:	
Cardiologist	Heart conditions
Rheumatologist	Arthritis and joint diseases
Neurologist	Neurologic problems
Nephrologist	Kidney problems

Gastroenterologist	Stomach irritations, ulcers, screening for colon cancer, colon polyp removal
Critical care	Intensive care
Endocrinologist	Hormonal abnormalities
Allergist	Allergies
Infectious Disease	Infections
Pulmonologist	Lung Diseases
Neurologic Surgeon	Brain tumor removal, slipped discs repair
Nuclear Medicine	Diagnose diseases by interpreting the image made by radioactive particles administered to the patient
Ophthalmologist	Eye surgery, laser treatments, infections
Otolaryngologist (ENT)	"Head and neck surgeons"; cancer removal, reconstructive surgery; treats dizziness; sleep apnea (tonsil removal), allergies, sinus problems

Oncologist	Cancer treatment with chemotherapy
Pathologist	Diagnose diseases via microscopic examination of tissue (biopsy)
Radiation Oncologist	Cancer treatment with radiation
Radiologist	Diagnose diseases via radiographic examination (x-rays, CAT scans, MRI)
Plastic Surgeon	Corrective surgery for apparent deformity
Preventive Medicine	Crisis prevention by analyzing data (epidemics, chronic diseases)
Psychiatrist	Treatment of mental conditions, often with medication
Orthopedic Surgeon	Removal of bone tumors, treatment of broken bones; treats distressed joints

Thoracic Surgeon	Treats lung and esophagus cancer; chest trauma; emphysema; lung transplants
Urologist	Medical and surgical treatment of bladder, kidney and adrenal glands; abnormalities of the male reproductive organ

Reviewing Table B shows that a specialist treats a specific condition while other specialists treat other conditions. Unlike primary care doctors who can treat multiple conditions, specialists focus on a particular condition and should not treat patients that do not have the condition that he/she specializes in. A specialist should not treat a patient that should be seen by a different type of specialist.

Specialists may also possess further expertise by taking yet additional years of training, called fellowships, after their specialty training. These doctors have "subspecialized" within their specialty. For a demonstration of this, please see Example 4, in this chapter.

Example 4. Basic Medical Knowledge: Who are Medical Specialists?
<u>Scenario:</u>

Specialist: Dermatologist
Subspecialty: Dermatologic Surgery

Discussion: A dermatologist is a doctor who specializes in the management of skin diseases. If it is determined that a patient needs a highly skilled skin surgeon to remove a lesion on a delicate, cosmetically important area like the eyelid, then a dermatologic surgeon could be suggested. Such a surgeon would have engaged in extra years of training in skin surgery. Therefore, this doctor is a specialist (dermatologist) with a subspecialty in dermatologic surgery.

Subspecialists also include specialists who have done additional training focused on a population defined by age. For example, an oncologist is a specialist that treats cancer patients with chemotherapy. A pediatric oncologist is also a cancer specialist but has additional training in cancer treatment in children. Such a specialist would be recommended to treat a child with cancer.

1.4   Who are Medical Extenders?

There has been a rise in medical extenders that practice some primary care, without being medical doctors. These include nurse practitioners and physician assistants. They may have their own practices, but are usually in a group under the direction of a medical doctor. These professionals are a part of the healthcare team and add another perspective to your treatment. For a variety of possible reasons, some patients may feel more comfortable relaying their problems to these professionals than to a doctor. (For more information on medical extenders, please see Chapter 2.2.2, Doctor Selection: Choosing a Medical Professional with the Best Training to

Treat Your Condition: Medical Doctor vs. Other Healthcare Professionals, and Chapter 9.2.1, Trends In Healthcare: Use of More Healthcare Professionals: Medical Extenders.)

1.5   What is Board Certification?
A doctor that has obtained board certification has spent years training in a chosen field (including primary care disciplines) and has passed a national examination. Doctors that are not board certified may or may not have completed the required number of years of training in a particular discipline or were unable to pass the written (and sometimes oral) national examination. These doctors may be just as skilled as their board certified colleagues but have not met the national board requirements. In many cases, HMOs (Health Management Organizations) will only list doctors that are board certified [3].

1.6   What is Alternative Medicine?
Alternative medicine is just that, an alternate form of medicine when compared to traditional medicine. "Alternative" refers to using a non-mainstream approach in place of conventional medicine"[4]. It involves non-traditional or non-conventional medical practices. Alternative medicine often lacks approved standards recognized by a national certifying agency.

Traditional (conventional) medicine, on the other hand, is the form of medicine that is standard for Americans. It is referred to as Western medicine and is based on allopathic medical principles. Allopathic principles use studies (case-based research) to devise methods to treat patients. The resulting treatment plans are taught in medical schools and other doctor training programs and are considered the standard of care. Allopathic medicine is further explained in Chapter 2.21, Doctor Selection: The Difference Between Medical Doctors: M.D. vs. D.O.

Although traditional medicine is the standard type of medicine practiced in the United States, many patients combine traditional medicine with alternative medicine treatments. As of 2014, nearly 40 percent of Americans, were not only using traditional medicine, but rather were also using healthcare approaches developed outside of mainstream Western, or conventional, medicine [4]. The combination of traditional and alternative medicine is called complementary medicine [4].

An example of complementary medicine (traditional and alternative medicine practices combined) would be if you saw a sports medicine doctor for traditional treatment (such as medication and physical therapy) but also used alternative medicine (such as routine massage).

Boundaries between complementary and traditional medicine overlap and change with time [4]. Using the same example from the previous paragraph, massage, once considered alternative, is used regularly in some hospitals to help with pain management. In this way, the inclusion of massage therapy into a treatment plan may not be considered alternative anymore.

The most widely used complementary products are natural products [4]. Natural products include herbs (also known as botanicals), vitamins and minerals, and probiotics [4]. "They are widely marketed, readily available to consumers, and often sold as dietary supplements: examples include, Echinacea, fish oil/omega, Ayurveda products (from India) and traditional Chinese medicine products (from China) [4].

The most widely used complementary services are mind and body practices [4]. Mind and body services that have become mainstream include meditation, massage, yoga and possibly acupuncture. Other mind and body services include traditional healers, homeopathy, and naturopathy [4]. But since these products and services are not apart of the Western medicine tradition and have not been studied to satisfy Western standards, such as by the Federal Drug Administration (FDA), an American physician may not choose to incorporate these products into a complimentary medical treatment plan.

Example 5. Basic Medical Knowledge: What is Alternative Medicine?

Scenario: A 48-year-old cyclist experienced excruciating lower back pain accompanied by reduced leg movement. A MRI showed a weak spinal ligament resulting in disc herniation and pressing on the spinal cord. The first doctor recommended that the patient have a series of steroid injections into the affected area to mask the pain. The patient obtained a second opinion from a different doctor after feeling uneasy about the first. The second doctor, on the contrary, suggested muscle relaxants, anti-inflammatory medication, physical therapy and if needed (PRP) platelet rich plasma injections, not steroids.

Discussion: The patient opted for treatment with the second doctor because that doctor offered complementary medicine (both traditional and alternative methods) to treat his condition. Muscle relaxants and physical therapy are examples of traditional medicine methods. Platelet rich plasma (PRP) is an example of alternative medicine. PRP uses the patient's own blood to heal and strengthen ligaments. Although there are currently no large research studies on the effectiveness of PRP, the risks associated with it seems minimal, in comparison to steroids. Long-term effects of steroid use, on the other hand, can be detrimental to one's health, and does not strengthen ligaments. If the patient had chosen the first doctor, the patient's condition could have worsened in time because steroids do not strengthen ligaments.

1.7 What is Integrative Medicine?

Integrative medicine combines traditional and non-traditional (alternative) medicine into one office location. In essence, it is a single location for complementary medicine. "For example, cancer treatment centers with integrative healthcare programs may offer services such as acupuncture and meditation to help manage symptoms and side effects for patients who are receiving conventional cancer treatments such as chemotherapy" [4].

Many individuals, healthcare providers, and healthcare systems are integrating complementary practices into treatment and health promotion [4]. "Driving factors include marketing of integrative care by healthcare providers to consumers who perceive benefits to health or well-being, and emerging evidence that some of the perceived benefits are real or meaningful" [4].

Scientific evidence of complementary medical products and practices is limited. "While there are indications that some may be helpful, more needs to be learned about the effects of these products in the human body and about their safety and potential interactions with medicines and with other natural products" [4].

Summary: Basic Medical Knowledge

- Ask your doctor what is your diagnosis and does he/she intend to treat your symptoms or diagnosis, or both.
- Choose the type of primary care doctor that best suits you and your family's needs. Each member of your family may be better suited with a different doctor, depending on the condition and age of the patient.
- Understand why a particular specialist should treat your symptom or diagnosis.
- There are other medical professionals (nurses, physician assistants) that are often directed, by a doctor, to treat you or prepare you for treatment.
- A board certified doctor has completed training and has passed the national examination for his/her discipline as required by the national examining board. A non-board certified doctor has not achieved both of these requirements.
- Some forms of alternative medicine are being used in conjunction with traditional medicine, for example the inclusion of massage therapy or acupuncture in a treatment regimen. The use of both alternative medicine and traditional medicine together is called complementary medicine. A treatment location that practices complementary medicine is called an integrative medical facility.

References

1. Centers for Medicare and Medicaid Services. Glossary-Referral. Retrieved in June 2013, from http://www.medicare.gov/glossary/r.html
2. Belsky, J (1984). *The Psychology of Aging: Theory, Research, and Practice.* Brooks/Cole Publishing Co.
3. New York State Department of Financial Services (2009). New York Consumer Guide to HMOS. Retrieved June 2013, from http://www.dfs.ny.gov/consumer/health/cg_hmo2009.pdf
4. National Center for Complimentary and Alternative Medicine. Complementary, Alternative, or Integrative Health: What's In a Name? Retrieved on March 24, 2014, from http://nccam.nih.gov/health/whatiscam

2

Doctor Selection

CHOOSING A DOCTOR CAN BE A daunting task. You could look through your medical insurance catalogue's list of doctors or search the Internet. You could also walk into a doctor's office that you have seen while driving by in your car. However, it is best to know something about your doctor before randomly choosing one. And although no method is perfect, all options are better than randomly choosing one. If possible, use multiple methods, that is, research the doctor before walking in.

2.1 Getting a Recommendation

2.1.1 From Someone You Know

One way to find a doctor is to take a recommendation from a friend, colleague, family member or another doctor. If you decide to ask someone to recommend a doctor, it is important for you to know and trust the person's opinion.

The trusted person (the recommender) who will make the recommendation should not be a person that you do not know personally. As a trusted person in your life, you should probably have an idea of his/her motivations, personal style and professionalism.

Although a doctor's accomplishments (publications, administrative rank, societal recognition, etc.) may be reasons to choose one doctor over another for your care, a recommendation from a person you know should carry as much weight in your decision. However, it is important that this person is a rational, intelligent person, as determined by your professional, personal and social experiences. In this situation, endorsement made by a trusted relative, friend, or colleague for a particular doctor, should be seriously considered. This is because thousands of doctors graduate from medical school every year, all with varying skills despite all of them passing their examinations. In other words, despite possessing an abundance of book knowledge, a doctor's ability to practice is dependent on his/her skill. Therefore, in order to decide which of the many doctors to choose from, advice from a trusted person can help you in reaching that decision.

A person's recommendation must be closely analyzed, or else your health may fall into the hands of a below-average doctor or a doctor whose skills may not be the best for you. Example 1, in this chapter, demonstrates this point.

Example 1. Doctor Selection: Getting a Recommendation: From Someone You Know
Scenario: A woman recommended a dentist (doctor of dentistry) to another employee. The employee needed a root canal and went to the "highly recommended" dentist. That dentist ultimately destroyed her nerves, leaving them open, raw and susceptible to infection.

Discussion: This example demonstrates the importance of determining the basis for the recommendation. The colleague had not seen this dentist for root canal but recommended the dentist because she and her children got annual cleanings from his assistant with an occasional cavity filling. Such procedures are vastly different from root canal. Therefore, the recommendation was not based on actual experience.

When asking for a recommendation for a doctor from someone whose opinion you trust, believe and understand, there are specific questions you should ask. The answers to these questions will help you understand why the person is recommending a particular doctor and whether that recommendation would be best for you and your condition. Questions that you should know the answers to before booking an appointment with a newly recommended doctor are as follows:

- How well do you know the recommender?
- What was the recommender's medical problem?
- Is the recommender's problem resolved?
  - If so, what was done? How long did it take?
  - If not, why would the recommender still suggest this doctor?
- Does the recommender personally know the doctor or know someone who knows the doctor personally?
- How did the recommender find this doctor?
- How long ago did this doctor treat the recommender?
- What other factors influence the recommender to suggest this doctor? Ex. Ease in obtaining appointments,

punctuality of appointment schedule, location of doctor's office, etc.

The motive for asking these questions should be clear. The point listed in #4 highlights that a recommendation may be given to you based on reasoning that could be irrelevant for the best treatment of your condition. Point #7 examines the proximity of the doctor's office. Keep in mind, that a doctor located around the corner from you may not be the best doctor for your condition.

A recommender may suggest a doctor to you that is comical or amusing. Although charm and wit are desirable traits for your doctor to possess, it is actually unimportant in relation to their medical skills. Of course, you may feel better when your doctor is personable and therefore, you may be more likely to follow your medical regimen, but the doctor's ability to tell jokes will not mask his/her actual skills. In other words, would you prefer to have your emergency appendectomy performed by a funny doctor with mediocre skills or by a no nonsense doctor with impeccable skills?

At the same time, a doctor with absolutely no interpersonal skills may create a negative environment. In such an uncomfortable environment, you may feel intimidated and not ask questions about your medical condition or give him/her a full description of your symptoms. And since there is some evidence to believe that your psyche or outlook may contribute to your prognosis, you should find a physician that feels like a comfortable fit [1].

Finally, when your doctor recommends another doctor, you still must question this referral. Although it may be awkward for you to ask your doctor, it is important for you to find out the relationship between these doctors. Of course, if you have had positive experiences with your doctor, it is plausible to assume that his/her recommendation is a sound one.

2.1.2 From Someone You Do Not Know

Some doctors advertise themselves in magazines, advertisements and even on the subway. Again, such sources may not give you full insight, as the doctors often pay for this publicity themselves.

Researching on websites that rate doctors also may not give you full insight about a doctor's skill. In fact, anyone can rank a doctor on some of these sites, including people that were never patients of that doctor. Some websites even include performance categories that do not apply to a specific doctor type, yet anyone that has Internet access can rank that doctor on an activity the doctor does not practice. Please see Example 2, in this chapter, as it demonstrates this point.

Example 2. Choosing A Doctor: Getting a Recommendation: From Someone You Do Not Know

<u>Scenario:</u> A radiologist is a type of doctor that interprets tests such as X-rays, MRI and CAT scans. These doctors usually do not meet with patients. Yet, an Internet search of a radiologist will display a bevy of rankings for this doctor.

<u>Discussion:</u> Some websites will have such a doctor ranked based on the doctor's interaction with patients (bedside manner) and the ease of obtaining an appointment with such a doctor. Clearly, such a ranking system would not apply to a doctor that does not see patients, such as a radiologist. Yet, a radiologist is graded based on such criteria. This demonstrates the questionability of Internet-based doctor rankings.

Even recommendations by celebrities may not apply to your situation. When a celebrity that you feel you share some commonality with recommends a particular cosmetic/medical product, you must realize that it may not pertain to your specific problem. Because you don't know that celebrity personally, you don't know his/her motivations; it is likely that the celebrity has a contract to endorse a product produced by a particular doctor and/or company. Additionally, the severity of your condition may differ from that of a celebrity. Finally, using a cosmetic/medical product advertised by an infomercial may worsen a separate condition of yours.

2.2   Choosing a Medical Professional with the Best Training to Treat Your Condition

Healthcare professionals include a wide variety of trained medical workers including, medical doctors, chiropractors, podiatrists, optometrists, psychologists and nurses. It is important for you to know the differences between healthcare professionals. Patients assume that all healthcare professionals are doctors with MD (medical doctor) degrees. This is not the case. The abbreviation after a healthcare professional´s name stands for the type of degree that the professional has.

There are various types of healthcare professionals who can legally treat your medical condition. These healthcare professionals should pass national examinations and show practical competence. In order to choose the type of professional that is best for you, you must choose the professional with the most certified training and experience in treating your condition. In order to do this, you must understand that the years of training, including exposure to certain diseases and their treatments, vary between these professions.

2.2.1 The Difference Between Medical Doctors: M.D. ("Medical Doctor") vs. D.O. ("Doctor of Osteopathy")

A doctor with a M.D. degree is one that has completed 4 years of training at an allopathic medical school. M.D. stands for "Medical Doctor". Allopathic medicine is taught at this type of school. Allopathic medicine is a Western approach to treating a patient after analyzing studies and other evidence-based treatment plans. It is the approach to medicine that is most popular in the United States and Europe.

A doctor with a D.O. degree is one that has completed 4 years of training at an osteopathic medical school. D.O. stands for "Doctor of Osteopathy". Osteopathic medicine is taught at this type of school. Osteopathic medicine is a holistic approach to treating a patient with an emphasis on alleviating the cause of the condition.

Allopathic medicine (M.D.) and Osteopathic medicine (D.O.) training in the United States is very similar. Both M.D. and D.O. doctors are medical doctors (physicians) that compete for the same residency programs (training after medical school) and can prescribe medication and perform procedures.

Unlike a M.D., a D.O. must obtain training in manual manipulation techniques. Manipulation (manual treatment) is a form of therapy in which a D.O. doctor uses his/her hands to relieve muscular and joint tension, throughout the body. To understand how this therapy differs from a chiropractor, please see Section 2.2.2, Medical Doctor vs. Other Healthcare Professionals: *Chiropractor vs. M.D.*, in this chapter.

Manual manipulation can be particular useful for patients suffering from pain due to neuro-musculoskeletal diseases. Manipulation learned during osteopathic training is unique to D.O. students. Traditional M.D. students do not learn this technique. This is important because manipulation can be successfully used as an alternate form of treatment for some conditions [2]).

2.2.2 Medical Doctor vs. Other Healthcare Professionals

Medical Doctor (M.D.) vs. Chiropractor (D.C.)
A certified chiropractor is a person who holds a D.C. degree. D.C. stands for "Doctor of Chiropractic" practices. Such a professional has studied neuro-musculoskeletal disorders, mostly originating from the spine for 4 years, at a Chiropractor College, A chiropractor focuses on disorders of the musculoskeletal system and nervous system [3]. Much emphasis is placed on spinal misalignment. Fixing this misalignment could cure the patient of a host of abnormalities. A chiropractor did not attend medical school and cannot prescribe medication or perform surgery [3].

The amount of training that a medical doctor, such as an orthopedic surgeon, neurosurgeon, neurologist and physiatrist, obtains beyond that of a chiropractor is extensive. Not only have these medical physicians completed 4 years of medical school, but they have also completed anywhere from 3-7 additional years of specialty training.

Medical Doctor (M.D.) vs. Podiatrist (D.P.M.)
A podiatrist has a DPM degree. This stands for "Doctor of Podiatric Medicine". A podiatrist is a foot doctor that is medically trained in diseases of the foot, ankle and lower leg.

These doctors perform surgeries, set fractures, fit orthotics and perform physical therapy. However, depending on your condition, a medical doctor (M.D or D.O.) with certification in Orthopedic Surgery and/or Dermatology may be better suited to treat a particular condition. For example, if major surgery is needed, an orthopedic surgeon may be your best option given the full body (above the leg) training that an orthopedic surgeon has undertaken. And although podiatrists are trained to recognize and treat skin and nail diseases of the foot, for complicated cases, perhaps a dermatologist would be better suited for your case, given the number of training years specifically dedicated to skin and nail diseases.

Medical Doctor (M.D). vs. Optometrist (O.D.)

An **ophthalmologist** is either a M.D. or D.O. In contrast, an **optometrist** is an eye doctor that is not a M.D. or D.O.

An ophthalmologist is a medical doctor (either M.D. or D.O.) that is certified by the American Board of Ophthalmology. Unlike an optometrist, an ophthalmologist can perform complicated and non-complicated surgeries and can recognize hundreds of eye conditions, in addition to writing prescriptions for eyeglasses and contact lenses.

An optometrist, on the other hand, has an O.D. degree. This stands for "Doctor of Optometry". An optometrist is an eye doctor who tests and treats patients for eye diseases and poor vision. They can prescribe medication and corrective eyewear. In some states, they are allowed to perform small surgeries and procedures such as foreign body removal, laser treatment and lacrimal/corneal injury therapy. These doctors often work in malls or national chain stores that sell eyeglasses.

Medical Doctor (M.D.) vs. Psychologist (Ph.D.)

A **psychiatrist** is a medical doctor that specializes in psychiatry and has a M.D. or D.O. degree. A **psychologist, on the other hand,** has a doctoral degree, but not a medical doctoral degree. A psychologist is a "Doctor of Philosophy" (Ph.D.) or a "Doctor of Psychology" (Psy.D.).

Both a psychiatrist and a psychologist will see a patient in need of behavioral assessment and/or behavior modification. A psychiatrist has completed four years of medical school, a year of general medical training and 3-4 years of psychiatric instruction. A psychiatrist, therefore, has knowledge about all diseases of the body, including psychiatric conditions and can prescribe medication. Therefore, treatment can involve the use of psychotropic drugs when seen by a psychiatrist.

On the contrary, a psychologist will spend on average 5 years after college, studying and conducting research on psychological entities. A psychologist cannot prescribe medication.

Both a psychiatrist and a psychologist undergo years of clinical training. Clinical training is training that involves patient assessment, diagnosis and treatment. A psychiatrist may work in an office/clinic or hospital setting. A psychologist, on the other hand, often practices in an office/clinic or school setting. Counseling and psychotherapy may be employed.

Treatment can vary depending on the severity of the mental condition. Thus, the nature of the patient's condition can dictate if a psychiatrist or a psychologist would be best suited. In some cases, the two professionals may work in unison to treat a patient.

Medical Doctor (M.D.) vs. Medical Extender
(Registered Nurse (RN), Nurse Practitioner (NP) and
Physician Assistant (PA))

A registered nurse (RN) is a nurse that has completed 2 years of nursing training and performs basic duties when encountering a patient (taking vital sign, etc). They usually cannot write prescriptions without a doctor's oversight.

A nurse practitioner (NP), on the other hand, possesses a master´s degree or DNP (Doctor of Nursing Practice) and in many cases can prescribe medication and perform small procedures. Some states require that a nurse practitioner work under a doctor's direction, others do not.

A Physician Assistant (PA) works under the supervision of a doctor and carries out the "plan" the doctor has written out, including prescribing medication and small procedures. (For more information on what a "plan" entails, please see Chapter 4.2.1, During The Medical Visit: Medical Documentation of Your Condition: The Medical (SOAP) Note, Subsection: Plan.)

2.3 What is an International (Foreign) Medical Graduate?

An international medical graduate, as labeled by the American Medical Association, is any student, American or non-American, who attends a medical school outside of the United States [4]. Therefore, an international medical graduate is an American who went to medical school outside the United States, or a non-American that went to a medical school in their own country or any other country besides America. These doctors were once called "foreign" medical graduates, but are now referred to as "international" medical graduates. Please see Example 3, in this chapter, for further details.

Example 3. Doctor Selection: What is an International (Foreign) Medical Graduate?

Scenario: An American financial advisor (of Russian descent) decided to go to medical school. She not only had the drive to leave her lucrative financial career, but to also complete pre-medical classes as an adult. Of the American medical schools she applied to, she was rejected from each one. However, a medical school in Greece accepted her. She moved to Athens in order to attend medical school. She is now an orthopedic surgeon, practicing in the United States.

Discussion: This scenario demonstrates the drive that many international medical graduates have to practice medicine in the United States.

Graduates of international medical schools that want to practice in the United States must take the same three national examinations administered by the United States Medical Licensing Board, that all students from American medical schools take. Generally, residency training (years of training doctors must complete after medical school) not done in the United States must often be repeated in the United States in order for these doctors to practice in the United States.

For you, a potential benefit in seeing a physician who completed residency training abroad is that this same physician generally repeats some portion of his/her training and/or schooling in the United States, in order to work in America. This means, that such a physician has spent nearly twice the amount of years training, before a patient can see them in the United States. (Please keep in mind that if their residency was completed in some European countries, namely Germany, Switzerland and England), these physicians may not have had to repeat all of their training.) Twice the training can yield twice the knowledge and experience before seeing patients in the United States. Even if the physician´s training was in a country where the most prevalent of diseases are rarely seen in the United States, it is still a benefit to the American patient as this physician has experience with the most common and rarest diseases and therefore may have a wider experience base to diagnose from.

2.4 The "Hidden" Doctor You "Cannot" Choose

A "hidden" doctor" is a doctor that does not actually see the patient he/she is helping. Despite this, such a doctor is a critical member of the medical team supporting the patient's health. Without meeting the patient, the "hidden" doctor helps determine the diagnosis and subsequent treatment of a patient.

A "hidden" doctor is a medical doctor that has completed the same 4 years of medical school as other M.D. or D.O. physicians. After completing medical school, the "hidden" doctor trains for 3-5 years in a specialty. Such specialties include pathology and radiology.

Most patients are unaware that a doctor, not chosen by them, is involved in their healthcare. Highlighted earlier in this chapter, Section 2.2 Choosing a Medical Professional with the Best Training to Treat Your Condition, is the importance of knowing the amount of training your healthcare professional has undergone. It is <u>critical</u> for you to have such knowledge of your "hidden" doctor's training as well.

Ask your doctor which "hidden" doctor will interpret your pathology or radiology tests and what their level of training is. If you are not satisfied with your doctor's responses regarding the training of the "hidden doctor", then ask for your test to be reviewed by another pathologist or radiologist. The act of having your diagnostic material reviewed by another doctor is called a consultation. You can ask your doctor to order a consultation (review) of your previously tested material. In this way, you will have a second opinion of your specimen or radiographic image. Be sure to check if your medical insurance will cover the cost of a consultation.

Pathologist

When a medical provider draws blood, collects urine, takes a biopsy or performs a surgical procedure, the specimen that has been removed is sent to a laboratory for interpretation. For liquid specimens, such as blood and urine, devices overseen by medical directors are used to determine the results. For non-liquid specimens, a pathologist will determine the results.

A pathologist is a medical doctor who specializes in diseases of the body on a cellular level. For tissue, the pathologist will examine your removed tissue under a microscope, determine a diagnosis, and send the diagnostic report to your doctor. Your doctor, or the doctor's staff, will then relay your diagnosis to you. Depending on the diagnosis, no further treatment, additional treatment or alterative treatment may be sought.

Empower yourself; request that your doctor send your specimen to a pathologist outstanding in his/her field, such as a board-certified, highly trained specialized pathologist. Example 4, in this chapter, highlights the importance of the "hidden" doctor's skills.

Example 4. Doctor Selection: The "Hidden" Doctor You "Cannot" Choose

Scenario: A patient had a small mass from her vagina removed by a dermatologist. After removing the mass, the dermatologist then interpreted the mass microscopically, instead of sending the mass to be read by a pathologist. The dermatologist diagnosed the tissue as completely benign. Consequently, nothing further was done for the patient. Five years later, the patient returned because the mass had grown substantially. At that time it was interpreted as cancer, by a board certified pathologist, with subspecialty training in skin. Because of the delay in diagnoses, the patient underwent two subsequent surgeries, radiation treatment and sustained fertility loss.

Discussion: The importance of the competence of the "hidden doctor" is truly exemplified in dermatology. If you have a biopsy taken in a dermatology office, your tissue could be examined by any of the following doctors:

- A dermatologist with little subspecialty training in pathology
- A pathologist with little subspecialty training in dermatology
- A dermatopathologist with subspecialty training in both dermatology and pathology

When diagnosing diseases on the microscopic level, it is best to have a doctor who has done advance training in microscopic diseases to interpret your results.

This example is not to say that a dermatologist without specialty training should not interpret biopsies (as it is legal and ethical for them to do so at this time), but for you to realize your power in deciding who will interpret your biopsy. It is up to you if you prefer someone who has had less training or not. The importance of this chapter is to emphasize that you have a choice, once you are empowered with the knowledge that these "hidden doctors" exist.

Radiologist
Likewise, when you have an x-ray, MRI or any other image of your body tested, ask your doctor about the skills/training of the radiologist that interpreted your test. Ask if the radiologist is board certified and has an outstanding reputation.

Summary: Doctor Selection
- Be cautious with any recommendation from family, friends, colleagues, doctors, the Internet, and advertisements.
- Consider the healthcare professional's expertise (M.D. or other training).
- Question your treating doctor about the expertise of the "hidden doctor" involved in your care.

References

1. Herrmann-Lingen, C., Klemme, H., & Meyer, T. (2001). Depressed Mood, Physician-Rated Prognosis, and Comorbidity as Independent Predictors of 1-year Mortality in Consecutive Medical Inpatients. *J Psychosom Res.*, Jun;50(6):295-301

2. Wolf C.J. (2008). Osteopathic Manipulation & Its Use for Low Back Pain. *Mo Med.*, 2008 Mar-Apr;105(2):163-7

3. American Chiropractic Association. (2013). What is Chiropractic?. Retrieved June 2013, from http://www.acatoday.org/level2_css.cfm?T1ID=13&T2ID=61

4. American Medical Association. (1995-2013). International Medical Graduates. Retrieved in June, 2013 from http://www.ama-assn.org/ama/pub/about-ama/our-people/member-groups-sections/international-medical-graduates.page

3

Preparation For The First Medical Visit

THERE ARE A FEW THINGS THAT you can do to facilitate your first office visit in order to get the most out of it. This chapter offers a few ways to accomplish this.

3.1 Planning for the First Medical Visit

Doctors are often impressed when their patients have knowledge about their own health. Having knowledge or showing interest in your health encourages the doctor, as your own enthusiasm excites him/her. The doctor will feel that you are now a part of the team, as opposed to a passive player. This will build a trusting, honest relationship between you and your doctor.

When seeing a new healthcare professional, be prepared to share your basic health history [1]. If you have a very complex health history, bring the names and addresses of your other physicians so that your new doctor can request records afterward if necessary [1]. Perhaps, make a list of questions to ask your doctor.

Regardless of your symptoms or condition, it is best to bring any medications that you have been taking or have previously taken, with you when you see a new healthcare professional. Knowing what type of medication you are using or were using in the recent past, is not enough because the dosage and intake frequency should also be correctly relayed to your new doctor. In order to avoid forgetting such crucial information, it is likely easier for you to simply bring all medication in their original prescription bottles to the first visit.

Even if you are taking medication for a seemingly unrelated condition or a non-prescription drug, it is important to inform your new doctor [9]. For example, some antibiotics that are only supposed to be used for a short time period can directly affect the effectiveness of other drugs that are being used for chronic conditions such as hypertension and diabetes. Thus, knowing what medications you are taking long term as well as short term can greatly affect your new doctor's choice of drugs for your case [2].

In addition to bringing the actual medication bottles to your new appointment you should also bring any medical journal/log you may have recorded. The medical journal/log will show your new doctor that you have taken your medication as previously directed [3]. Sometimes, a doctor will choose to prescribe a particular medication based on a patient's reliability to take the medication as recommended. If a patient has shown that he/she may not reliably take his/her medication as prescribed, a doctor may opt to prescribe a drug that requires less compliance and less frequent dosing [4].

Be sure to bring any other health related journal/log to your initial office visit, not just the medication log. This can include diet and/or exercise logs. Such information can be useful for your new doctor as it gives your new doctor a clearer picture of you. Your doctor may even be able to offer you guidance [5].

If you have copies of any medical tests or medical reports relevant to your visit, you should bring these documents as well. In this way, a doctor may opt not to repeat a study if he has evidence that you have already had it done. Such documentation includes laboratory reports and radiographic images/reports. If you do not have a copy of these items, just having knowledge of where you had the study performed can aid your new doctor in retrieving this information, if necessary.

Thanks to advancements in technology, electronic medical records are resulting in patients not having to carry their medications, logs and previous tests results to each new doctor visit. (Please see Chapter 9.1, Trends In Health Care: E-Health.) But until electronic medical records are universal, you should still bring these items with you.

3.2 Overcoming Barriers to Care

Although you may encounter problems that challenge your access to healthcare, never let anything prevent you from obtaining it. Problems can range from simple to extremely complex. Table C lists some barriers to healthcare and potential solutions. If you experience a barrier other than what is listed, find your own means to overcome it. Never give up; seek help from others if you are unable to solve the problem yourself. Ask family and friends for advice, check government websites and perhaps hire a lawyer. Examples 7-12 from Chapter 5.5, After The Medical Visit: Getting Help From Family, Friends and Organizations, demonstrate how others can help you to overcome barriers.

Table C.
Overcoming Barriers to Care

Barrier	Solution
No Health Insurance	Contact www.healthcare.gov for guidance
Language	1. Contact your doctor's office and request that the office provide a service that can translate during your visit. There are interpretation services that the office can engage. 2. Take a trusted translator with you to the visit. This translator could be a family member or friend.
Cultural/ Social	1. Do not be shy! Inform your doctor about how your culture influences your view of medicine. This includes your cultural attitude towards medication, treatments, and physical examinations. Failure to inform your doctor of your cultural beliefs could result in failed treatment of your condition. (Please see Chapter 4.2.1, Example 4.) 2. Your doctor may have taken "cultural competency" training courses.

Non-Emergency
Transportation

Financial   The doctor's office may be able to help facilitate transportation money via donation programs if you qualify. For example, The Cancer Society of America may have some money available for those suffering from life threatening cancer that are unable to reach the treatment facilities because of a lack of money.

Disability   If you are eligible based on your disability and other guidelines, major cities such as New York City have door-to-door transportation services for a small fee, such as Access-A-Ride. Search on the Internet for similar services in your town by using key words like: transportation services to doctor's appointment

Too Few Doctors
In Your Town   1. Telemedicine may or may not be an option, depending on your circumstance, and likely requires a local doctor/hospital to access. (Please see Chapter 9.2.2)

2. You may need to travel

| Limited Education | Ask your doctor to take the time to explain your concerns and to refer you to information centers and services that could aid you. |

Summary: Preparation For The First Medical Visit

- Have some knowledge about your previously diagnosed condition.
- Write down concerns about your health and share these thoughts with your doctor.
- Bring a list of your previous healthcare professionals.
- Bring all medication bottles.
- Bring all health related journals/logs.
- Bring your medical reports/images.
- Ask your doctor for advice to overcome a potential barrier.
- Request contact information for agencies or companies that can aid in serving you.

References

1. One Medical Group. (2011, May 11). Take Note: 7 Ways to Optimize Your Next Office Visit. Retrieved from http://www.onemedical.com/blog.

2. U.S. Department of Health and Human Services. Your Medicine: Be Smart. Be Safe. (With Wallet Card). Agency for Healthcare Research and Quality. Retrieved in May 2013 from http://www.ahrq.gov/patients-consumers/diagnosis-treatment/treatments/safemeds/yourmeds.html.

3. American Academy of Family Physicians. Creating a Health Journal. Retrieved June 2013, from http://familydoctor.org/familydoctor/en/healthcare-management/working-with-your-doctor/creating-a-health-journal.html.

4. Brown, M.T. & Bussell, J.K.Medication (2011). Adherence: Who Cares?. Mayo Clin Proc. April; 86(4): 304-314.

5. Waggle, S. Reviewed by Forresster, J. 10 Tips for Sticking to Your Diet. *Ladies Home Journal.* Retrieved May 2013, from http://www.lhj.com/health/weight-loss/keeping-weight-off/10-tips-for-sticking-to-your-diet/

4

During The Medical Visit

WHILE AT THE DOCTOR'S OFFICE, THERE are actions you can take to better your medical experience. The most important is probably being honest and open with your doctor regarding your health. Such honesty will foster a stable relationship with your doctor and allow for him/her to offer you the best care possible.

4.1 Ways to Build a Positive Relationship with Your Doctor

When meeting a doctor for the first time, do not feel wary or skeptical. Doctors are people who have taken an oath to help others. Most doctors genuinely want their patients to get better and are eager to assist them upon meeting them.

It is normal to feel nervous, embarrassed and apprehensive. However, keep in mind, that doctors have experienced a wide range of medical cases before seeing you. What is most important is that feelings of embarrassment do not prevent you from revealing all of your symptoms and concerns. Example 1, in this chapter, emphasizes this point.

Try to remain calm. If you are too anxious, your blood pressure will be elevated at the time of recording your vital signs. Although your doctor is busy, he/she wants to learn about your condition so that the best treatment plan for you can be devised. So, feel free to be yourself and express your concerns.

You can also relay to your doctor how you found him/her. Doctors feel appreciated and validated when they learn that someone recommended them. Finally, follow the doctor's orders.

Example 1. During The Medical Visit: Ways to Build a Positive Relationship with Your Doctor

Scenario: A mother brought her baby to a hospital clinic because the baby had a cough and fever. The examination was near completion when the doctor figured that the infant had a common cold. Just as some of the staff walked away from the baby, the mother quietly stated that the baby was HIV positive.

Discussion: Such a condition greatly effects the possible treatment options for the infant because patients with HIV are more likely to catch particular colds as opposed to some other common types. If the mother remained too afraid to divulge that her baby was HIV positive, her baby would have been treated in a different manner initially. This would have delayed the baby from receiving optimal care.

4.2 Medical Documentation of Your Condition

4.2.1 The Medical (SOAP) Note

Your conversation with your doctor is filtered and transcribed, by the doctor, into what is called a SOAP note. SOAP is an acronym that represents the four categories of the note; Subjective, Objective, Assessment and Plan [1]. The information obtained during your conversation with the doctor is entered into the note under one of the four categories. The SOAP note outlines the pertinent medical issues in a systematic way, so that any other medical professional can easily interpret the doctor's notes. It can ultimately be used to track your medical history. In other words, the SOAP note organizes the conversation between you and your doctor including the treatment plan, for each visit. In essence, the SOAP note is a progress report documenting your condition.

The SOAP note is composed of all the information a doctor gathers about you during the office visit, and also documents the doctor's plan to treat your condition. This allows any medical professional to easily read and assess your condition and progress, without having to review information in a random fashion [2]. The SOAP note also provides the doctor with a structured guideline when conducting the office visit and forces the doctor to enter information that may have otherwise been inadvertently missed.

Your chart is composed of SOAP notes from each visit, as well as other medical information such as laboratory results [2]. Therefore, if you request a copy of your medical chart, you will receive the notes from each visit, which should be written in the format of a SOAP note for each visit. Some doctors, especially those that have practiced for some time, may not write out the headings for each category of the

SOAP note, but all of the information that would be in the SOAP note would still be included [2].

It is important to understand that each of the four categories generally elicits information that the doctor must obtain in order to complete the note. This is why a doctor asks probing questions at the office visit, for the doctor must fill out the SOAP note. The SOAP note forces a doctor to be systematic in his/her questioning and be rational in his/her approach to treatment.

Subjective Section (SOAP)
The first category of the SOAP note is the Subjective section of the medical note. This section is simply a recording of your view of your own condition and reason for the visit [2]. Thus, it is critical to recognize that the Subjective section of the note is your personal feelings, not the doctor's feelings, about you or your condition. In fact, the doctor should never record his/her personal feelings about you, unless it is substantiated by medical evidence. In other words, a doctor should never have a simple feeling about you or your condition, but instead must have a medical opinion.

In the Subjective section, the doctor records your reason for the visit. If this is your first visit with the doctor, then the Subjective section of the SOAP note is generally much longer and inclusive, than future notes. This is because your family history, medical (clinical and surgical) history, social history, current medications and allergies are recorded in this section at the time of the first visit. This information as a whole is referred to as the History of Present Illness [2]. The word "history" is used to denote that the information includes data from the past.

The information elicited from the Subjective section of the SOAP note is very important. Here is a detailed explanation of what can be revealed:

Chief Complaint - This is the main component of the Subjective section. The chief complaint is your reason for going to see the doctor. It is the main reason for the visit. For example, the chief complaint cannot merely be a headache. Instead, it must be qualified to explain the reason why you came in at that very moment. So, if your visit is due to a headache, the chief complaint could be "the worst headache of your life" or a "persistent headache". By qualifying the headache, the doctor or any other medical professional reading the note will understand the reason for your visit.

Family History - This information provides the doctor with important clues for the genetic and social risk factors of your current, past and/or future condition. Neglecting to inform a doctor about a family illness could result in a delay of diagnosis for you. For example, informing a doctor about your strong family history of cancer could result in earlier detection of cancer for you, as screening for specific genetic cancers are recommended at an earlier age than the general public.

Medical History- This information provides the doctor with findings regarding your current condition and includes facts from your past medical conditions. It is important to be as inclusive as possible when relaying the information from years past regarding your medical history. Informing the doctor of seemingly non-relevant illness in the past, may contribute to the doctor's overall opinion regarding your current state. Without relaying the full medical history, you jeopardize an accurate and timely diagnosis with treatment.

Included in the medical history, is a list of all past surgical procedures and treatments. For example, rushing into your doctor's office or emergency room complaining of severe abdominal pain on the right side will elicit from the doctor a long list of possible causes, including a ruptured appendix. Not informing the doctor that your appendix was removed twenty years ago could waste potential life-saving time, because the unknowing doctor may spend time considering a ruptured appendix as the source of the pain.

Social History - This information provides the doctor with an idea of your behavior and risk factors for current or future illness. This information includes your smoking, drinking, exercising and sexual practices. In this section, illegal drug use is also explored.

The use of herbs and natural agents must also be revealed. Some patients will take these agents for deep-seeded religious and/or cultural beliefs. Some of these agents are fine, but others may block the effectiveness of the medical drug that the doctor has prescribed. Dr. Barrie Cassileth, chief of the Integrative Medicine service at the Memorial Sloan-Kettering Cancer Center, states

"A common, false belief is that 'if it's natural, it must be safe...But herbs and other dietary supplements are biologically active compounds, and they frequently have negative interactions with prescription pharmaceuticals." [3]

For this reason, it is important for the doctor to be aware of any herb or natural agent ingested by the patient. Examples 2-4, in this chapter, demonstrate the importance of providing accurate social information to your doctor.

Example 2. During The Medical Visit: Medical Documentation of Your Condition: The Medical (SOAP) Note

Importance of the Social History

<u>Scenario 1:</u> A 67-year-old male patient had been a chronic alcohol abuser since he was a teenager. He failed to inform the doctor of this, despite the doctor asking him if he drank alcohol. Because the patient had already had a heart attack, the doctor prescribed a blood thinning medication to reduce the patient's likelihood of developing a stroke. The doctor was unaware of the patient's long history of alcohol abuse.

<u>Discussion:</u> Alcohol abuse can reduce the liver's ability to clot blood. Not informing the doctor of chronic alcohol use while taking a blood thinning medication, could lead to uncontrollable bleeding.

Example 3. During The Medical Visit: Medical Documentation of Your Condition: The Medical (SOAP) Note

Importance of the Social History

Scenario 2: A 59-year-old man began taking an herb thinking that this "natural" agent could benefit him during his cancer treatment.

Discussion: Some patients may ingest "herbal" mixtures concocted in a non-regulated setting. This includes herbal remedies purchased at health stores, herbalist shops and Eastern medicine/Alternative holistic centers. It is important that a doctor obtain this information, while interviewing the patient, as side effects or a negative interaction with a prescribed drug, could occur. For example, some experts believe that garlic extract, St. John's Wort and Echinacea could interfere with the effectiveness of some chemotherapy drugs used to treat cancer [3].

Example 4. During The Medical Visit: Medical Documentation of Your Condition: The Medical (SOAP) Note

Importance of the Social History

Scenario 3: A 29-year-old Asian woman went to her gynecologist for a breast exam. Although she was wearing a gown, the assistant in the room caught a glimpse of the patient's back. The assistant informed the doctor of unusual marks on the patient's back. The doctor asked the patient if he could see her back. The patient complied and the doctor saw many coin shaped red and purple bruises. He assumed that the patient was a victim of domestic abuse and confronted her about his concern. The patient explained that the marks on her back represented an important Vietnamese traditional method to treat illness.

Discussion: The patient had not been physically abused. She had used "...coining or "*Cao gio*", a form of dermabrasion commonly used in Southeast Asian cultures to rid the body of "bad winds" by bringing bad blood to the surface" (4,5). "*Cao gio* involves applying ointment to the skin and using a coin or spoon to firmly rub the skin until petechial or purpura appear" (5). "The result is a distinct, symmetrical pattern of bruises typically on the back, shoulders, chest, temples, and forehead that resolve without residual effects" (5). This scenario highlights how a doctor from a different culture can misinterpret and misdiagnose a traditional cultural practice. This exemplifies the importance of informing your doctor of religious/cultural practices.

Current Medication List - This list provides the doctor with critical information. You may be taking medication that is causing your symptoms or impairing the recovery of a different ailment. Example 5, in this chapter, demonstrates the importance of revealing your medication.

Example 5. During The Medical Visit: Medical Documentation of Your Condition: The Medical (SOAP) Note

Importance of Revealing Current Medication
Scenario: A patient saw a doctor for an ear infection and was instructed to take amoxicillin for 10 days, but experienced no relief after taking this medication for 5 days. The patient decided to see a different doctor on day 6.

Discussion: If the patient fails to tell the new doctor that he/she has been on amoxicillin for 5 days, the doctor may prescribe the same regimen that the previous doctor prescribed. This is because doctors are taught to treat certain conditions with first line drugs initially, and when this fails, then to prescribe a second-line drug. If, on the other hand, the patient informs the doctor that he/she has been taking amoxicillin, as prescribed by another doctor, for the last 5 days with no relief, the second doctor may recommend completing the trial of amoxicillin for a total of 10 days. The second doctor may then recommend that the patient return to his office, if relief does not occur after completing the treatment. Completing a drug regimen as prescribed by your doctor not only offers the greatest likelihood of recovery but also, in the case of antibiotics, may reduce your body's ability to become resistant to that drug for future infections.

Allergies- You must inform your doctor of your allergies. This information allows the doctor to safely prescribe new medication. Example 6, in this chapter, reviews this concept.

Example 6. During The Medical Visit: Medical Documentation of Your Condition: The Medical (SOAP) Note

Importance of Revealing Your Allergies

Scenario: A patient knew that she was allergic to penicillin but did not inform her new doctor because after examining her ear infection, the doctor told the patient that he would prescribe cephalexin for her infection.

Discussion: Studies have shown that patients allergic to penicillin may also be allergic to cephalexin. The patient could experience severe reactions secondary from taking this drug. (In reality, the doctor in this scenario should ask if the patient is allergic to penicillin before prescribing cephalexin.)

Objective Section (SOAP)

Unlike the Subjective section, the Objective section does not include a description of your condition in your own words. Instead, in the Objective section, your doctor will describe your condition using medical evidence, not your opinion. The Objective section, therefore, is non-biased information regarding your condition.

Non-biased information includes your vital signs (blood pressure, temperature, heart and respiratory rates), physical measurements laboratory and radiographic results [2]. When abnormal, these findings objectively signify to the doctor that something is wrong.

Objective findings may also include a previous doctor's assessment of your condition. Although this may seem subjective to you, a doctor's opinion is medically based and, therefore, should be considered objective.

Other Objective information to be recorded in this portion of the note is the all-important physical examination, conducted by your doctor. The doctor's physical examination is based on Review of Systems. The Review of Systems is quite simply when the doctor checks for normalcy starting from your head (testing of the eyes, ears, nose and throat) and finishing after examining more or less the entire body. Tests performed during the physical examination include listening to the lung and heart sounds, checking joint reflexes and observing the skin for any changes.

Doctors obtain very valuable information from the physical examination. They are not merely checking for signs of the ailments that you described in the Subjective section of the visit, but are also checking for the normalcy of your other body parts [6]. Examples 7 and 8, in this chapter, highlight the usefulness of the doctor's physical examination of you.

Example 7. During The Medical Visit: Medical Documentation of Your Condition: The Medical (SOAP) Note

Importance of the Doctor's Physical Examination of You
Scenario 1: A patient came to the office complaining of visual changes. During the eye examination, the doctor

was able to suspect diabetes, without first performing a blood glucose (sugar) level.

Discussion: The physical exam, or eye exam in this case, provided medical evidence of suspected diabetic changes. This finding would be recorded in the objective section of the SOAP note.

Example 8. During The Medical Visit: Medical Documentation of Your Condition: The Medical (SOAP) Note

Importance of the Doctor's Physical Examination of You
Scenario 2: A patient was seen for a cold, but upon performing a complete physical examination, the doctor found a suspicious mole.

Discussion: Although the patient came in for a cold, the doctor took the time to look over the patient's skin while performing the physical examination. A suspicious mole was noticed. The doctor removed the mole and sent it to the pathologist. The pathologist diagnosed the "mole" as melanoma, a malignant condition. The patient was subsequently treated for the melanoma. If the doctor did not find this melanoma when performing the physical examination, the patient may have developed metastatic disease that has a much shorter life expectancy. This finding would be written in the Objective section of the SOAP note.

Assessment Section (SOAP)

The Assessment section of the SOAP note is a declaration of all of the integrated findings from the previous sections, namely the Subjective and Objective sections. This declaration is the conclusion drawn by the doctor after reviewing all of the information. Within the declaration is the differential diagnosis. The differential diagnosis is a list of possible medical conditions that could be the cause of the patient's problem.

Thus, the Assessment contains the differential diagnosis for your case. Because multiple diseases can present with similar symptoms (subjective findings) and physical changes (objective findings), the doctor must include in list form, all of the possible causes for your case. This differential diagnosis is often listed with the most likely condition topping the list down to the least likely one [2]. (Please refer to Chapter 1.1, Basic Medical Knowledge: Symptom vs. Diagnosis, for further information on symptoms and diagnoses.)

The differential diagnosis list may change as you return for future visits. This is because as you follow your doctor's recommendation there may be full recovery, improvement or worsening of your condition. With this new information, the doctor will then write a new assessment for you with a more limited differential diagnosis and a more specific treatment plan. Of course, some symptoms are so specific that the doctor will not have a differential diagnosis and will only have a single diagnosis.

Plan Section (SOAP)

The Plan section of the SOAP note is the last entry for the progress note. This section is a description of how your doctor intends to treat your condition. It is the layout of how your doctor plans to restore you to good health. It is in this section that your doctor writes his/her medical recommendation as discussed with you. This recommendation may include sending you for laboratory tests, radiographic imaging, medications, surgery and/or referrals [2]. In this section, your doctor also records when you are to return for a follow-up visit and therapy recommendations, such as physical therapy [2].

4.2.2 Importance of Documented Accuracy

The notes taken by medical professionals are very important because those notes will stay with you for the rest of your life. Accuracy of your medical note, therefore, is essential. If a mistake is written in your note, it follows you forever. If a diagnosis, for example, is assumed, but never proven, but recorded anyway, it follows you.

Therefore, it is essential that you require that your doctor record accurate data about your history and your condition [7]. When you attend a doctor visit, you discuss your ailment with your doctor, but are probably not concerned about the accuracy of your doctor's recorded notes. However, to prevent possible problems in the future, it is best to ensure that your doctor records exactly what you have experienced, nothing more or less.

The importance of having accurate medical notes is not only exemplified by insurance company denials based on erroneous notes, but also in being able to track the onset of a disease. Since some diseases develop suddenly, while others slowly progress, a poor recording of your symptoms will make it difficult to determine when a particular disease may have actually started. Please see Example 9, in this chapter, for further details.

Medical students are taught that their medical notes are legal documents. This means that anything a doctor writes in your chart can be used in a legal proceeding sometime in the future [7]. This is a profound notion for a young doctor to comprehend. It basically means that what is written will be reviewed by others and the doctor is legally bound to what he/she has written. Therefore, young doctors are informed of this and are told to never remove a note from a chart.

A doctor removing a note from your chart makes the doctor appear guilty of making a mistake. Many medical-legal cases have been settled simply because the doctor went back to the chart and attempted to alter what was previously written. Even if the doctor was trying to add valuable, medically correct information to the note, the perception may be that this doctor is adding information to "cover up" a mistake.

Of course, sometimes, a doctor actually will remove or add information to a chart with the purpose of "covering himself/herself". This is another reason for you to ensure accurate medical notes are written on your behalf. This is difficult for a patient, being that patients generally lack medical knowledge and cannot validate medical data. Therefore, at the very least, requesting a copy of your medical note after each visit, will allow you to have your own log of your notes. (This would be recommended if you have a serious condition.) Thus, if any notes "disappear", you have evidence otherwise. (This topic is also discussed in Chapter 8.1, Medical Fraud and Medical Malpractice: Identifying Medical Fraud.)

Requesting a copy of your notes will also let your doctor know that you are aware of your medical care and that you are attentive to it. This should not be construed as aggressive, but rather as concern for your own health. Doctors appreciate patients that are engaged in their own healthcare

[8]. These patients tend to follow the doctor's recommendation, which is fulfilling for a doctor whose mission it is to see his/her patient's health improve.

Example 9. During The Medical Visit: Medical Documentation of Your Condition: Importance of Documented Accuracy

Scenario: A radiologist examined a patient's MRI of the brain. The radiologist found changes in the patient's brain that implied old age and also identified a suspicious mass in the patient's brain. This record was released to the patient's primary care doctor. The primary care doctor immediately called the radiologist to verify the findings given that the patient was only 20 years old with no symptoms of old age. The radiologist reviewed the MRI, to find that the wrong interpretation was recorded for that patient. However, because doctors generally do not remove previous notes from a patient's chart, the radiologist refused to remove the wrong diagnosis from this patient's chart. Instead, the radiologist wrote an addendum (second note) to the previous wrong one clarifying that the patient was actually healthy and had no mass lesion or senile changes.

Discussion: Since the second note clarifies the previous erroneous one, the patient should have no problems with insurance. However, this example demonstrates two things: 1) patients must review their medical notes for accuracy and 2) doctors often catch the errors of other providers and act as check points for the entire process. In this way, medical errors are often caught before damage occurs to patients.

Summary: During The Medical Visit
- Build a positive relationship with your physician by being honest, showing interest in your health and following your doctor's orders.
- Medical documentation of your condition
    - Be sure to provide your doctor with all information requested about your medical and social history.
    - Ensure that your medical notes (SOAP) and records are accurate.

References

1. Soap Note. 2013, January 11. Sample Notes: All About Writing Notes and Samples. Samplenote.org. Retrieved 2013, December from http://www.samplenote.org/soap.html.

2. Physician Soap Notes. Retrieved June 2013, from http://www.physiciansoapnotes.com

3. Reynolds, S. Dietary Supplements and Cancer Treatment: A Risky Mixture. National Cancer Institute. Aug 11, 2009 (9) 16.

4. Davis RE. Cultural Health Care or Child Abuse? The Southeast Asian Practice of Cao Gio. *J Am Acad Nurse Pract*. 2000 Mar;12(3):89-95.

5. Harris, TS. Bruises in Children: Normal or Child Abuse? *J Pediatr Health Care*. 2010;24(4):216-221. Retrieved on 2013, November 29 from Medscape Multispecialty.

6. Bloomfield, H.E. and Wilt, T.J. (Oct 2011). Evidence Brief: Role of the Annual Comprehensive Physical Examination in the Asymptomatic Adult. Evidence-based Synthesis Program (ESP) Center, Minneapolis VA Medical Center. Bookshelf ID: NBK82767PMID: 22206110. Retrieved June 2013, from http://www.ncbi.nlm.nih.gov/books/NBK82767/

7. Gorney, M., Jenkins, P.A., Dixon, L.A., & Shepard S. (2003 & 2008). Accurate Medical Records: Your Primary Line of Defense. The Doctors Company. Retrieved June 2013 from http://www.thedoctors.com/KnowledgeCenter/PatientSafety/articles/CON_ID_000318

8. Wantland DJ, Portillo CJ, Holzemer WL, Slaughter R, McGhee EM. The Effectiveness of Web-based vs.

Non-Web-Based Interventions: A Meta-analysis of Behavioral Change Outcomes. J Med Internet Res. 2004 Nov 10;6(4):e40. Retrieved from http://www.jmir. org/2004/4/e40/v6e40. doi: 10.2196/jmir.6.4.e40.

5

After The Medical Visit

AFTER YOUR MEDICAL VISIT, YOU ARE left with many options to consider. You will start by examining your feelings about the visit. Hopefully, you trust the doctor and understand the purpose of his/her treatment recommendations. Perhaps you have been inspired to learn more about your condition. Alternatively, you may decide that the visit did not meet your expectations and therefore, may opt to end the relationship with this doctor. Regardless of your decisions, this chapter reviews the many options you will likely consider after your medical visit.

5.1 Decisions to Make

5.1.1 Do You Like/Trust Your Doctor?

Regardless of whether your doctor is new to you or familiar, the patient must decide whether or not to continue the patient-physician relationship. It is the patient, not the physician, who makes this decision. (Albeit, a physician can terminate the patient-physician relationship under certain circumstances [1].)

Upon leaving the physician's office, regardless of the diagnosis, you should feel like you are in good hands. Trusting your physician is beneficial to your health for many reasons [2]. Firstly, it creates a positive relationship between the two of you. Such a relationship fosters a more open discussion of your condition, which could lead to providing the doctor with useful clues about your treatment plan. Secondly, trusting your doctor will likely result in better patient compliance with your treatment plans [2]. Thirdly, by trusting your doctor, you reinforce the notion that you believe in his/her expertise. This affords your physician positive feedback and will make him/her more relaxed when seeing you.

Alternatively, if you do not trust your doctor you have to figure out why and to what extent [3]. If you are doubtful about your physician's abilities, it is best to obtain a second or third opinion [4]. If, on the other hand, you completely do not trust your physician, then it is best to consider a new relationship with a different physician.

Let's say that you decide to see a second physician because you completely disregard the opinion of the first. Unfortunately, you also feel that the second doctor has not warranted your trust. At this point, you may opt to see a third or fourth physician. You must shop for a doctor and obtain multiple opinions until you feel comfortable with one [4].

Your ultimate goal is to feel that you can trust your doctor. Until that is accomplished, you will never feel confident that your condition is being optimally treated [2,3]. Examine your instincts, if you do not trust a doctor, even if the doctor is a world expert in his/her field, perhaps you do not trust him/her because you do not understand your condition, or perhaps the doctor seems rushed and does not spend enough time with you. These reasons could create a feeling of distrust, however, this does not mean that you would not receive the best care from this doctor [3]. Therefore, it is important for you to examine your feelings; ask yourself, "what is behind this feeling of mistrust"? Do not let frivolous reasons get in between you and having the best care by a great doctor. If a doctor performs well, but you feel is condescending towards you, perhaps addressing your feelings with him/her directly is the best approach. By clearing up uneasy feelings, you may develop a trusting relationship with your doctor.

5.1.2 Do You Understand the Treatment Recommendation?

After you have found a doctor that you trust, you may be confused by the doctor's treatment recommendation. In order to relieve this anxiety, you should ask your doctor to explain the purpose of each treatment [5]. By sharing with you the goal of each treatment, you will understand your condition better [5]. In this manner, you become empowered against your condition because you know exactly what the treatment is combating [5].

Perhaps a treatment recommended for you by your doctor involves using medication that you do not want to take. Again, you must ask your doctor specifically how a particular medication works to fight against your ailment. You then must weigh the benefit of the medication against your own feelings about taking such medication, not to mention documented side effects. Your doctor may be able to offer a suggestion that would require you to take less medication. For greater understanding of this option, please see Example 1, in this chapter.

Example 1. After The Medical Visit: Decisions to Make: Do You Understand the Treatment Recommendation?

Scenario: In order to reduce the frequency that a patient needed to take pain medication for spastic muscles, the patient opted to take occasional warm baths with Epson salt.

Discussion: Instead of relying on pain medication completely, this patient discussed with her doctor some other tactics that could be utilized to reduce her pain. Ultimately, she had to continue with her pain medication but she was able to reduce the frequency in which she had to take them because the warm baths helped reduce the pain.

If you decide that you still do not want to take a particular medication, ask your physician for an alternative medication or treatment [5]. Unfortunately, there may be no other proven treatment option.

If you decide not to take a recommended medication or if you stop taking a medication that you were once taking, you must inform your doctor [6]. This gives him/her the opportunity to find other options for you immediately. Under no circumstances should you stop taking your medication without notifying your doctor. Failure to notify your doctor could result in irreversible damage. Example 2, in this chapter, emphasizes this point.

Example 2. After The Medical Visit: Decisions to Make: Do You Understand the Treatment Recommendations?

Scenario: A 60-year-old man who had been on anti-hypertensive medication for many years decided to stop taking his medication as he developed a suspicion for any drug he was ingesting. Unfortunately, he had a stroke within a week of stopping his medication.

Discussion: The anti-hypertensive medication had been used to prevent a stroke (which he had not fully understood). He subsequently became paralyzed on one side of his body. A year later, he lost his balance and fell. In doing so, he broke his leg. His leg was then set improperly, resulting in an amputation above his knee.

If he had continued to take his anti-hypertensive medication or at least told his doctor that he was no longer planning to take the medication, perhaps this domino-effect would have been prevented.

If further testing is recommended...

Be sure to understand your treatment recommendations. Further testing such as blood work and radiographic imaging provides doctors with the ability to make a diagnosis with certainty. As long as you trust your doctor and you have asked what the purpose of the test is, testing should be performed.

5.1.3 Do You Understand the Purpose of a Referral?

If your doctor refers you to another doctor, there should be a medical reason for it. You must ask why you are being referred and what is the goal of the referral. Because medicine has become more complex, primary care doctors refer their patients to specialists and subspecialists seen as experts in the latest treatments [7]. It is your job to ask why you are being referred, upon which receiving the answer, may provide you peace of mind and also continued trust of your doctor. Examples 3 and 4, in this chapter, demonstrate how referrals can benefit your health.

Example 3. After The Medical Visit: Decisions to Make: Do You Understand the Purpose of a Referral?

Scenario: Perhaps your doctor recognizes that you have been afflicted with terrible health news, but after a year, you are still emotionally suffering from the diagnosis and you are unable to carry on with your normal functional living routines.

Discussion: At this point, your doctor may recommend that you see a psychiatrist to help you to sort out your feelings and perhaps prescribe and monitor anti-depressive medication. Your instinct may be to not see the psychiatrist and even get offended by your doctor's referral. However, seeing a psychiatrist may actually help you to fight, and ultimately, overcome your ailment.

Example 4. After The Medical Visit: Decisions to Make: Do You Understand the Purpose of a Referral?

Scenario: A 23-year-old man had stretched a ligament in his wrist. His doctor prescribed physical therapy. The young man did not think that physical therapy was important and therefore did not attend.

Discussion: The young man should have asked his doctor how physical therapy would help his condition. He would have learned that this form of therapy would not fix the ligament but it would build strength of the surrounding muscles to help compensate for the stretched ligament. Armed with such details, he may have been convinced to participate in physical therapy activities, as he would now understand how it could benefit his overall condition.

If a specialist is recommended...

When a doctor suggests that you see a specialist, it is for your best interest. Your doctor wants to see you well and therefore will send you to other medical professionals who can help facilitate this. If a doctor is unable to cure you on his/her own, he/she will seek additional, outside advice and help to treat you.

As with any treatment plan, be sure that you trust the new medical professional in order to get the most out of your experience. This is best accomplished by asking many questions about your treatment plan and overall health.

5.2 Understanding Your Condition

Once you are made aware of your diagnosis, you can ask your provider for a pamphlet explaining it in further detail. Researching your condition online as a non-medical person could result in misunderstanding your condition and lead to panic. If, however, you choose to research your diagnosis on the Internet, be sure to ask your doctor, at the next visit, about what you read. Your doctor is equipped with the knowledge to tell you what is true and what to disregard [8]. In this way, any misinterpretation on your part can be cleared up.

Examples of Conditions You Can Research

If possible and if you are interested, you can learn about your condition to a degree that you can truly understand it. After learning about your condition to this degree, you may be able to visualize what therapy would be needed to correct the problem. For some patients, this is very useful; to know exactly what is wrong may reduce a level of anxiety [9]. Others may not want to know exactly what is wrong [9].

Example 5, in this chapter, exemplifies the level of detail in which you can learn about a condition. The goal is to be able to actually visualize the impairment so that you can also visualize how the treatment can target the problem and correct it. Keep in mind that self-diagnosing is **never** recommended.

Example 5. After The Medical Visit: Understanding Your Condition

<u>Scenario:</u> A woman, who had never suffered from acne as a teenager, developed it in her mid-thirties for the first time. Although it was likely due to hormonal changes, the clinician began the woman's acne treatment with a benzoyl peroxide cleanser. After a few months of minimal improvement, an antibiotic was added. Again, after minimal improvement, an additional therapy was added to the regimen. Finally, after a year of trying different therapies, the doctor considered prescribing the strongest medication to combat acne. However, this medication could have serious side effects, including liver damage and could cause significant fetal defects. Regardless, the patient opted to take this medication and signed a contract stating that she agreed to have periodic liver tests and to avoid pregnancy while on this medication.

<u>Discussion</u>: In this scenario, acne is the condition that this patient may choose to research further with the help of her doctor. If she did, she would learn the following:

Acne, most commonly seen in teenagers, is the blockage of pores that lead to dirt, oil, and bacteria build up, under the skin [10]. The blockage can be due to a variety of factors including hormonal changes (puberty, pregnancy, menstrual cycle, menopause, medication), humidity, make-up and unclean skin [10].

Figure 5.1 shows a normal pore. Figure 5.2 shows a pore affected by acne. In Figure 5.2, there is a proliferation of oil (sebum), likely due to blockage of the pore (for the reasons mentioned in the previous paragraph). As a consequence to the increase in oil development and pore blockage, the number of bacteria will grow. (Notice that the normal pore also contains some bacteria.) Bacteria flourish as they eat the abundant oil. The straight hair arising from the normal pore bends and breaks. The broken hair and bacteria attract inflammation. Inflammation is the cause of the red and white skin color changes seen in acne and is a hallmark of the gradual destruction of the pore. This inflammatory process causes the skin to slightly elevate in this area, forming a pimple, as seen in Figure 5.2. This is a recurrent process unless something is done to break the cycle.

Figure 5.1   NORMAL PORE

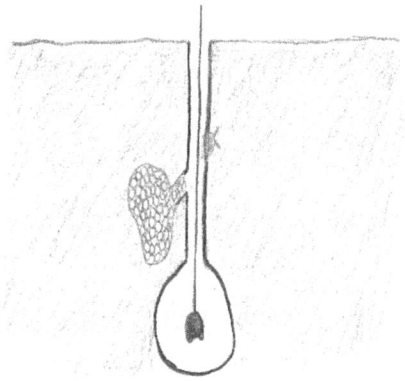

KEY

This image shows a normal, narrow pore with a hair shaft growing straight up and out onto the skin surface. There is one bacteria on the right side of the pore and is identified by the "v" shaped antennae.

Figure 5.2   ACNE PORE

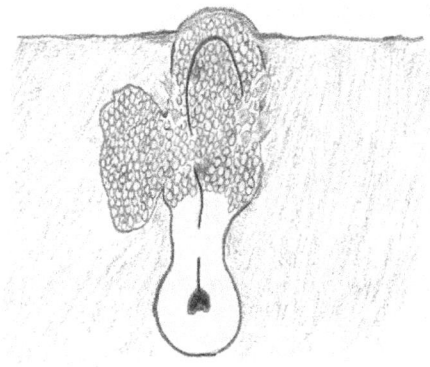

Key

This image shows a pore with acne: broken hair shaft, proliferation of sebum oil (balls) and bacteria with accompanying inflammation. The surface shows a slight dome shaped elevation, which is the pimple.

If untreated and allowed to proliferate, more pores undergo this transformation and eventually each will explode under the surface of the skin, as the pore is unable to hold the oil, bacteria, broken hair shaft, and inflammation. Consequently, more inflammation occurs under the skin leading to broad cyst development and scar formation overtime.

By understanding how acne develops as described above, the patient can then ask the doctor how each ingredient in the prescribed treatment regimen will work to destroy the acne. The patient is empowered. The doctor can now explain the treatment as such:

Treatment is aimed to break this cycle by keeping skin clean, reducing oil production, and killing the bacteria. If you are prescribed benzoyl peroxide, its purpose is to kill the bacteria. If you are given antibiotics, its purpose is to kill stubborn bacteria. An anti-inflammatory ingredient, such as salicylic acid, is used to reduce the overall inflammation and to clear up the clogged material within the pore. This will significantly decrease the redness and bumps seen in acne lesions. If your acne becomes overly dry while treating it, your body will produce more oil. This will result in more production of bacteria, as the oil serves as food for the bacteria. Therefore, an ingredient is added to your regimen to prevent drying out your acne too much. Hormonal therapy targets excessive oil production by also decreasing oil production and therefore reduces the bacteria food supply. Finally, the last line of treatment against acne is a medication that has been known to cause fetal abnormalities and is therefore not prescribed to women who are pregnant or considering pregnancy. Patients on this drug must agree to routine blood test to if the patient is male or female.

Please see your doctor for further details about preventing, detecting and treating acne; do not try to self-diagnosis.

5.3 Getting a Second Opinion

Americans today are taking more responsibility for managing their own health by seeking second opinions [11]. A second opinion means you are consulting with another doctor to confirm a diagnosis and/or find possible different treatment choices available to you [12]. It is your right as a patient [11, 12]. In fact, it is recommended to get a second opinion immediately to avoid delays in your treatment and recovery [12].

Second opinions are a way for a patient to learn about his/her diagnosis [12]. Understanding your diagnosis is critical in deciding your choice of treatment [12].

"For minor health problems, second opinions are usually unnecessary. However, a second opinion is probably a good idea if you are:

- Having major surgery
- Questioning whether surgery is the only option
- A problem that has been difficult for your regular doctor to diagnose
- Having trouble talking to your current doctor(s)

- Not seeing improvement in your medical condition
- Diagnosed with a life-threatening disease such as cancer, heart disease or brain tumor
- Told a second surgery is recommended
- Having multiple medical problems" [11]

Although second opinions may be awkward for you to initiate and for the doctor to accept, studies have shown that 30 percent of patients, who sought second opinions for elective surgery, found that the second opinion was different from the first opinion [12]. Additionally, 18 percent of patients who were required to obtain a second opinion by their insurance company found that the two opinions were not in agreement [12]. Example 1, from Chapter 8.1, Medical Fraud And Medical Malpractice: Identifying Medical Fraud, demonstrates the positive consequences of getting a second opinion.

"Keep in mind that doctors are human and they too can make mistakes or be faced with unusual or challenging cases" [12]. "Because of the increase in medical knowledge and new treatments, it is difficult for any one physician to be aware of all the latest information" [11]. "A different doctor may come up with a different diagnosis, or at least offer a different opinion as to treatment choices. Factors which may have an effect on a doctor's opinion are technology available to that doctor, school of thought, where they were trained, individual methods of treatment and experience in dealing with that particular diagnosis" [12]. Also, some doctors are more conservative while others tend to be more aggressive [12].

When getting a second opinion, if the first doctor's opinion is the same or similar to the second doctor's, you will feel reassured [12]. If, on the other hand, the second doctor doesn't agree with the first, you may feel unsure of what to do [13]. "In that case, you may want to talk more about your condition with your first doctor or talk to a third doctor" [13]. As previously stated in this chapter, Section 5.1.1, Decisions to Make: Do You Like/Trust Your Doctor?, if you do not trust your physician, then it is best to consider a new relationship with a different physician. You must shop for a doctor and obtain multiple opinions until you feel comfortable with one [4].

Example 6. After The Medical Visit: Getting a Second Opinion

Scenario: Ten years ago, a 55-year-old man attended a routine doctor's visit. A blood test showed elevated cholesterol. The doctor recommended for this otherwise healthy patient to start taking a cholesterol-lowering medication. The patient was surprised to learn of his high cholesterol and consequently opted for a second opinion. The patient got a copy of his blood test and brought it to a second doctor. The second doctor reviewed the laboratory work and stated that the patient did not need to take a cholesterol- lowering drug and that it was the patient's "good" cholesterol that was elevated. (Elevated "good" cholesterol is helpful to your health.)

Discussion: The patient's "good" cholesterol was elevated, not the "bad" cholesterol. Perhaps the first doctor misread the laboratory result and thought the "bad" cholesterol was elevated. Regardless, ten years later, the patient has never taken a cholesterol-lowering drug and has a normal, healthy cholesterol blood level. Had the patient not opted for a second opinion, he would have taken the cholesterol-lowering drug unnecessarily and could have been subjected to negative side effects from the medication.

Once you have decided to get a second opinion you must decide how to go about it. One option is to ask your doctor for the name of another doctor [13]. This is a difficult option to choose as you may not feel comfortable telling your first doctor that you are seeking a second opinion. "A good doctor understands your right to be well informed and should support a second opinion" [12]. "Ask your doctor to send your medical records to the doctor giving the second opinion" [13]. "Be an informed consumer and arrive for the second opinion with all of your previous medical records, contact information about the first physician, insurance card, list of prescribed medications and allergies, and any diagnostic test results" [12]. "That way, you may not have to repeat the tests you already had. Also, call the second doctor's office and make sure they got your records" [13].

A second option is to ask a different doctor you trust to recommend a doctor [13]. This option allows you to obtain a recommendation from another healthcare professional without having to ask your first doctor for it.

The third option is to find a second doctor on your own. If you do not tell the second doctor that you previously saw another doctor, it is called a "blind second opinion". "The advantage of the blind second opinion is that it cannot be influenced by previous information. The disadvantage is that your second opinion doctor may not be able to tell you why his/her opinion is different without knowing the basis of the first doctor's opinion" [11].

Below are questions to ask during a second opinion appointment:

- "Is there a chance the medical problem could have a different diagnosis?
- Are there any alternative forms of treatment available?
- What are the likely results if you wait or don't have the treatment?
- What are the risks associated with the treatment(s)?
- Are there any side effects or residual effects from each treatment option?
- How is the treatment plan expected to improve your health or quality of life?
- How long is the recovery period?
- If the second opinion differs from the initial one, why? (It is important to understand the reasoning behind a medical opinion.)" [11]

"Second opinions may be mandatory for certain conditions or procedures" [11]. In fact, your insurance or health plan may reduce or eliminate the benefits paid if a second opinion is not obtained [11]. Assuming a secondary opinion is medically necessary, most insurance plans will pay for at least part of the cost while Medicare will pay 80% of the cost [12]. "As a matter of fact if the second opinion doesn't agree with the first, Medicare will pay 80% of the cost of a third opinion. Patients that belong to a Medicare Health Maintenance Organization (HMO) are entitled to a second opinion, but some plans require a referral from your primary care physician, and like most HMO treatments, you must see an in-network physician" [12].

Most second opinions are voluntary but may still be paid for by your insurance or health plan [11]. "[A]lways check with your insurance or health plan for specific policies" [11]. Call your insurance provider before going for any treatment or second opinion to prevent any confusion or denial of the bill. You need to know exactly what will be covered, such as an out-of-network provider, any lab work or testing that may be required and what your responsibilities are before seeking the second opinion [12].

5.4 Ending the Relationship with Your Doctor

If you feel that for whatever reason you have not had a favorable medical experience, you can decide to no longer maintain a relationship with that doctor's office. As stated in this chapter, Section 5.1.1, Decisions to Make: Do You Like/Trust Your Doctor?, a physician cannot abandon you, but you can opt to abandon the physician [1].

Once you have made this decision, you could request a copy of your medical records. The office is obligated to release this information to you. Having this information may be of benefit for the next provider you choose.

Doctors are allowed to end a patient-physician relationship under specific guidelines only, otherwise they can be charged with abandonment [1]. A doctor, for example, can recommend to the patient that the patient be seen by another healthcare professional. However, if the patient does not agree to take up care with the other professional, the original doctor should continue to see this patient.

Before deciding to "drop" your doctor, please review from this chapter, Section 5.1.1, Decisions to Make: Do You Like/Trust Your Doctor?, to be sure that you are doing what is best for you.

5.5 Getting Help From Family, Friends and Organizations

No man is an island; therefore, all men and women will need help from others at some point. Whether you obtain help from family members, friends or organizations, the support will be greatly needed. Depending on the diagnosis and treatment, a patient may need both medical and social support.

5.5.1 Medical Support

Depending on your situation, you may need assistance with your medical treatment. Examples 7 and 8, in this chapter, show the importance of obtaining medical support at home.

Example 7. After The Medical Visit: Getting Help from Family, Friends and Organizations: Medical Support

Scenario: A 40-year-old single woman decided to undergo fertility treatment. She would need to self-administer daily hormonal injections at home. She was afraid of needles and felt that she could not administer these injections herself. A college friend who happened to be a nurse, agreed to give her the daily injections.

Discussion: This scenario demonstrates how a family member or friend could help the patient with their medical treatment and ultimately relieve potential stress for the patient. Family and friends can help the patient with their medical care, including getting to appointments.

If you need assistance, but do not get it, your health maybe compromised. In this case, the lack of assistance could become a barrier to care. As described in Chapter 3.2, Preparation For The First Medical Visit: Overcoming Barriers to Care, you must find a way to solve a potential barrier to your care.

Example 8. After The Medical Visit: Getting Help from Family, Friends and Organizations: Medical Support

Scenario: An 82-year-old woman with multiple medical conditions and on many medications was found dead in her bed at home. The police found numerous medication bottles on the nightstand table next to her bed. An autopsy showed that she had died from toxic levels of a heart medication. The amount found in her body well exceeded the prescribed amount. Oddly, the other medications on the nightstand table, which were potentially more dangerous when taken in excess, were not found in her blood. In other words, a drug that is less toxic is the one that killed her...suggesting, that this was not a suicide, but rather an accidental death by administering the wrong medication.

Discussion: This woman took the total amount of medication, from one bottle, instead of taking the recommended amount from each bottle. If this woman had a caregiver, friend or family member to schedule her medication intake, she would not have mistakenly ended her own life.

If you do not have a family member or friend available to help you, you should inform the doctor to give you clearly written home instructions. Regardless of how much experience a doctor has treating a particular condition, for the patient, it is likely a new experience. And since many doctors seemingly "rush" through appointments, you should require written home instructions, tailored for your individual need. This may not necessarily be a pre-made pamphlet, but rather, instructions specifically for you. Some hospitals have a phone number that discharged patients can call to hear their home instructions, as often as they want and at anytime. Example 9, in this chapter, emphasizes the need to have clearly written home instructions for treating your medical condition.

Example 9. After The Medical Visit: Getting Help from Family, Friends and Organizations: Medical Support

Scenario: A 65-year-old man was to have eye surgery for a retinal detachment. The doctor verbally gave the pre and post homecare instructions. Immediately after the surgery, the doctor repeated the homecare treatment and sent the patient home. Among the many instructions given to the patient, one included keeping his head down for 8 hours out of the day, not including the sleeping hours. When the patient arrived home, he took a nap and upon waking up thought that the doctor had told him to keep his head down as much as possible, but not for the majority of the day. It seemed impossible to keep one's head down nearly all day.

Discussion: If the patient had a family member or friend to receive the instructions from the physician after surgery, perhaps that person would have more accurately remembered the homecare instructions. In this scenario, the doctor's office should have given the patient written home care instructions and informed him (before the surgery) of the various at-home devices that he could have used to keep his head down in a more comfortable way. These devices are often covered by insurance and are delivered and picked-up from the patient's home. Ultimately, the patient's eye did not heal at the rate it was supposed to, as the patient had not kept his head down.

5.5.2 Social Support

Depending on your situation, you may need assistance with your medical treatment. Example 10, in this chapter, demonstrates the importance of obtaining social support from a neighbor.

Example 10. After The Medical Visit: Getting Help from Family, Friends and Organizations: Social Support

Scenario: A 30-year-old male needed to have an outpatient procedure performed within the next week but did not have anyone to pick him up after the procedure. The doctor's office would not perform the treatment unless the patient had arranged for someone to pick him up afterwards.

Discussion: The doctor's office postponed the patient's procedure until the patient had identified a guardian for the day. A neighbor agreed to participate in such service.

If you need assistance, but do not get it, your health maybe compromised. In this case, the lack of assistance could become a barrier to your care. (Chapter 3.2, Preparation For The First Medical Visit: Overcoming Barriers to Care, lists solutions to other potential barriers to care.)

Having a family member or friend who can support you socially through this difficult time is priceless. Organizations like churches, synagogues, neighborhood councils and other societies may offer such support.

There are various types of organizations that could help if you do not have family or friends to assist you. To find out about such programs, ask your doctor during your visit. Your doctor will likely ask you to get details from the medical receptionist at the front desk. The receptionists may have pamphlets and other recommendations for you. Please see Examples 11 and 12, in this chapter, for further demonstration.

Example 11. After The Medical Visit: Getting Help from Family, Friends and Organizations: Social Support

Scenario: A 79-year-old woman living alone with complications of severe, untreated rheumatoid arthritis was in need of a meal but was in too much pain to go shopping.

Discussion: Not only could a family member or friend bring food to her, but she could also order food from a local grocery for delivery. Other alternatives include the use of programs for the elderly.

Example 12. After The Medical Visit: Getting Help from Family, Friends and Organizations: Social Support

Scenario: A 54-year-old woman with colon cancer needed to see her radiation oncologist for weekly radiation treatments. Her daughter attended the sessions with her. In order to get to these appointments, they took the bus. The patient attended the appointments at the beginning of each month because that is when she received her social security check and, therefore, had money to pay for transportation. However, by the middle of the month, the patient did not attend her radiation treatments as she had spent all of her money by then. Although her daughter served as her caregiver, her daughter did not have access to transportation. Both women lived below the poverty line. A medical assistant in the doctor's office learned of this patient's lack of money to get to her appointments. The medical assistant contacted a national cancer society to ask if there was a transportation scholarship/stipend that this patient could obtain. The society used money raised from its fundraising efforts to support this patient's efforts to attend her doctor's office.

Discussion: Radiation oncology, like other fields in medicine, require for the patient to commit to a highly regimented and scheduled treatment course. By missing appointments, the cancer is able to spread and grow. This defeats the purpose of treatment and also wastes money that has already been spent on previous appointments.

There are companies that help patients arrive at their office appointments. However, for various reasons, some patients may not qualify for such services. When this occurs, there are non-profit organizations, such as cancer societies, support groups and other agencies that might provide aid. As a patient in this position, you may need to search for such organizations on your own. Search the Internet or ask your doctor's office for a list of societies and other organizations involved in patient support for your particular condition.

Summary: After The Medical Visit
- Decisions To Make
  - Do you like/trust your doctor?
  - Do you agree with treatment recommendations?
  - Do you understand the purpose of a referral?
- Understand Your Condition
  - Talk with your physician.
  - Ask for a pamphlet explaining your condition.
  - If you decide to do some research of your own, keep in mind that you are not a medical professional and must ask your doctor to go over the information that you have found. Self-diagnosing is never recommended!
- Second opinions are important! You will learn more about your condition and treatment options. Do not hesitate to get one. Be sure to check with your insurance carrier if a second opinion will be covered.
- If you feel dissatisfied, end the patient-physician relationship with your doctor.
- Be proactive in seeking additional help from family, friends and local social/religious organizations.

References

1. American Medical Association. (2013) Ending the Patient-Physician Relationship. Retrieved June 2013, from http://www.ama-assn.org/ama/pub/physician-resources/legal-topics/patient-physician-relationship-topics/ending-patient-physician-relationship.page

2. Pearson, S.D., & Raeke, L.H. (2000). Patients' Trust in Physicians: Many Theories, Few Measures, and Little Data. *J Gen Intern Med,* July; 15(7): 509–513. doi: 10.1046/j.1525-1497.2000.11002.x

3. Mascarenhas, O.A.J., Cardozo, L.J., Alfonso, N.M., Siddique,, M., Steinberg, J., Lepczyk, M. & Aranha, A.N.F. (2006). Hypothesized Predictors of Patient–Physician Trust and Distrust in the Elderly: Implications for Health and Disease Management. *Clin Interv Aging.* June; 1(2): 175–188.

4. Ham, B. Seeking a Second…or Third…Opinion. Center for Advancing Health. Retrieved Retrieved June 2013, from http://www.cfah.org/prepared-patient/prepared-patient-articles/seeking-a-secondor-thirdopinion#.UY6Sp5WVg9c

5. Marcus, M.B. (2010, sept 1). More Empowered 'Patients Question Doctors' Orders. *USAToday.*

6. Cleveland Clinic. *General Medication Guidelines.* Retrieved June 2013, from http://my.clevelandclinic.org/healthy_living/medications/hic_what_you_need_to_know_about_taking_your_medications.aspx

7. Abelson, R. (2012 Jan 23). Doctors Refer More Patients to Specialists. Retrieved from http://prescriptions.blogs.nytimes.com/2012/01/23/doctors-refer-more-patients-to-specialists/

8. Diaz, J.A., Griffith, R.A., Ng, J.J., Reinert, S.E., Friedmann, P.D. & Moulton, A.W. Patients' Use of the Internet for Medical Information. (2002). J

Gen Intern Med. 2002 March; 17(3): 180–185. doi: 10.1046/j.1525-1497.2002.10603.x

9. Shattner, A. What do Patients Really Want to Know?. Oxford Journals Medicine QJM: An International Journal of Medicine Volume 95, Issue 3. Pp. 135-136. Retrieved June 2013, from http://qjmed.oxfordjournals.org/content/95/3/135.long

10. Berman, K. (Reviewer). Acne. (2012 Nov 20). *PubMed Health*. Zieve, D., Eltz, D.R., Slon, S. & Wang, N. (Eds). Retrieved June 2013, from http://www.ncbi.nlm.nih.gov/pubmedhealth/PMH0001876/

11. UK HealthCare. Getting a Good Second Opinion: Americans and the Second Opinion. From http://ukhealthcare.uky.edu/publications/healthsmart/getting-a-good-second-opinion/on 3/27/14.

12. PAF. Patient Advocate Foundation. Retrieved 2014, March 24 from http://www.patientadvocate.org/index.php?p=691

13. Medicare.gov. Getting A Second Opinion Before Surgery. Retrieved 2014, March from http://www.medicare.gov/what-medicare-covers/part-b/second-opinions-before-surgery.html

6

Medical Insurance: What To Know

IN ORDER TO LIVE A HEALTHIER and longer life, access to healthcare is critical. Now more than ever, many diagnostic and preventative services are free for members of a medical insurance plan. After the implementation of the Affordable Care Act, more Americans and their families gained access to the United States healthcare system.

6.1 Importance of Medical Insurance

Every person gets sick at some point; it is inevitable. Healthcare costs are incredibly expensive when there is no insurance coverage to pay off some of the expense. Without medical insurance, fixing a broken leg could cost as much as $7,500, and a three-day hospital stay could average $30,000 (1). People without coverage may become bankrupt or develop deep debt due to medical expenses [1]. For these reasons, the United States government mandated that every citizen have health insurance by 2014.

Besides offsetting bankruptcy or deep debt, health insurance may offer free preventive care. Vaccines, screenings, and check-ups may all be offered for free under your plan [1]. Thus, a mammogram or colonoscopy could be covered 100 percent by your insurance. Additionally, some costs of prescription drugs may be covered [1].

6.2 The Motivation of Medical Insurance Companies

Medical insurance companies are for-profit companies. They must generate money, not lose money, to stay in business. In order to keep investors, the bottom line must show annual profits. Every time medical insurance companies pay a claim, that is money subtracted from their bottom line. However, given the nature of the business, they must pay some claims.

The Affordable Care Act (ACA), also referred to as "ObamaCare" or The Marketplace, was not medical insurance or a medical insurance company. The goal of the Affordable Care Act (ACA) was different from that of the private medical insurance companies. The goal of the ACA was to "provide affordable, quality health care for all Americans and reduce the growth in health care spending" [2].

The ACA's motivation was to reduce the national healthcare spending by ensuring that everyone has health coverage that includes free preventative services. In the long run, disease prevention should reflect in a decrease in healthcare spending. Such motivation is very different from that of medical insurance companies.

Because of the ACA, medical insurance companies can no longer deny applicants based on the applicant having a pre-existing condition. This forces these companies to accept applicants who maybe more likely to have numerous medical bills. The insurance company can expect to lose money from their bottom line when having such a member (patient) on their plan.

However, the ACA also generates money for these companies because millions of Americans who did not have insurance before, will now join these companies as members. Each member brings money to the company because each member is required to pay numerous fees. The list of potential member fees include:

1. Premium- is the fixed cost of a member's insurance plan [1].
2. Deductible- a sum of money you must pay out of pocket before the insurance company will begin to pay some or the entire bill [1].
3. Copayment- "[a] copayment is a fixed amount you'll pay for a medical service after you've met your deductible. For example, after meeting your deductible you may pay $25 for a visit to the doctor's office that would cost $150 if you didn't have coverage. The health plan pays the rest" [1].
4. Coinsurance- is a fixed percentage you pay for a medical bill. "For instance, you may pay 20% of the cost of a $100 medical bill. So you would pay $20 and the health plan would pay the rest" [1].
5. Out-of-pocket maximum- is the total amount (deductibles, coinsurance, and copayments) you'll have to pay, each year, if you get sick [1]. The plan will pay for any covered care above that amount for the rest of the year [1].

The overall healthcare system (private and governmental) is expected to benefit from these new members because some of these people did not pay for health insurance previously. Before the Affordable Care Act was enacted, many individuals would live their lives, uninsured and were most vulnerable to developing debt and bankruptcy when an accident/emergency occurred. For example, these individuals would go to the emergency room, if they developed a bad cold. This, in turn, would drive up national healthcare costs, as the cost of an emergency room visit could be as much as 3 times more than a visit to a doctor's office. By requiring uninsured individuals (and every other American citizen) to have health insurance, more money is added to the healthcare system.

Thus, with new members come new fees that are collected by the medical insurance companies. This represents a new source of income for these companies. By admitting more members, the overall healthcare system obtains money by collecting membership fees. Their gamble is that the fees received outweigh the payments the companies must pay on behalf of these new members when they get sick. The overall projected benefit is to reduce national healthcare costs.

6.3 Type of Medical Insurance

6.3.1 Private Medical Insurance

Private medical insurance is coverage by a health plan provided through an employer or union or purchased by an individual from a private health insurance company [3]. There are numerous private medical insurance companies such as Aetna, Blue Cross Blue Shield, HIP, United Healthcare, Emblem, etc [4]. *Group medical insurance* and *individual medical insurance* and are both types of private medical insurance.

Group Medical Insurance

Group Medical Insurance is a group health plan offered as an employee/union benefit. It is established or "maintained by an employer or by an employee organization (such as a union), or both, that provides medical care for participants or their dependents directly or through insurance, reimbursement, or otherwise" [5].

"COBRA provides certain former employees, retirees, spouses, former spouses, and dependent children the right to temporary continuation of health coverage at group rates. This coverage, however, is only available when coverage is lost due to certain specific events" [6]. Group health coverage for COBRA participants is often more expensive than health coverage for active employees, since usually the employer pays a part of the premium for active employees while COBRA participants generally pay the entire premium themselves [6]. Insurance through COBRA is ordinarily less expensive, though, than individual health coverage [6]. Please see the next Section, *Individual Medical Insurance* for further information.

Individual Medical Insurance

Individual Medical Insurance is "a type of health policy that an individual purchases for himself and/or his family. Individual health insurance policies are often purchased with the guidance of an insurance agent to help navigate plan choices and premium costs" [7].

6.3.2 Government Medical Insurance

Government health insurance includes plans funded, by government, on the federal, state, or local level. The major categories of government health insurance are Medicare, Medicaid, the Children's Health Insurance Program (CHIP), military healthcare, state plans, and the Indian Health Service [3].

Medicare

Medicare is the federal program that helps pay healthcare costs for people 65 and older and for certain people under 65 with long-term disabilities [3]. A Medicare recipient is not automatically entitled to every benefit offered by Medicare [8]. Entitlement/coverage benefits depend on which provisions someone would qualify under [8]. The standard Medicare reimbursement is 80% of the allowed amount [8].

If you have two forms of insurance: Medicare and private insurance, Medicare is often primary and private insurance is secondary. But to confirm this, call your private insurance company and refer to your Medicare information booklet [8].

If, in fact, Medicare is deemed primary, it means that Medicare must analyze your doctor's bill first and determine the amount Medicare will pay towards that bill. If Medicare does not pay the entire bill, then the secondary insurance will review the remaining expenses. From there, the secondary insurance may pay some, if not all, of the remaining expenses.

Members that have both Medicare and private insurance must see doctors that take Medicare. They can no longer go to a doctor that does not take Medicare, even if that doctor accepts their secondary insurance. However, there are some circumstances in which Medicare can be bypassed and you can use your secondary insurance only. Such circumstances involve the need of specialty care that is not offered by a doctor that accepts Medicare. Please see Example 1, from this chapter, for a demonstration of this.

Example 1. Medical Insurance: What To Know: Type of Medical Insurance: Governmental Insurance: *Medicare*

Scenario: Due to a new disability, a 35-year-old woman was placed on Medicare but was also entitled to private insurance through COBRA from her previous job. Consequently, she had two medical insurances: Medicare (primary) and private insurance (secondary). Despite her disability, at this age, she needed fertility testing and treatment if she was to have a child. She found a facility that would honor her secondary insurance, but not Medicare.

Discussion: This patient was allowed to see a fertility specialist and get treated, while being covered by her secondary insurance. Medicare was never used, despite it being her primary insurance. This exemplifies one of the few occasions when Medicare (primary insurance) can be bypassed and the secondary insurance was used to cover expenses.

Medicaid

Medicaid is a program administered at the state level, which provides medical assistance to those in need. Families with dependent children, the aged, blind, and disabled who are in financial need are eligible for Medicaid. It may be known by different names in different states [3].

If you qualify for Medicaid, you will not qualify to participate in The Marketplace. Please see Example 2, from this chapter, to better understand this policy.

Example 2. Medical Insurance: What To Know: Type of Medical Insurance: Governmental Insurance: *Medicaid*

Scenario: A 45-year-old man, earning approximately $12,000 a year, attempted to sign up for medical insurance through The Marketplace in 2014. He worked part-time and therefore was not entitled to medical insurance through his employer.

Discussion: After applying for eligibility to participate in The Marketplace online, he was notified that given his income, he was not eligible to participate in The Marketplace in 2014. However, by applying to The Marketplace he found out that he did qualify for Medicaid. He subsequently applied for Medicaid and began receiving medical benefits shortly thereafter.

State-Specific Plans

Some states have their own health insurance programs for low-income uninsured individuals. These health plans may be known by different names in different states [3].

6.4 Appealing a Denied Claim

If your medical insurance company refuses to pay a bill that you feel they have an obligation to pay, appeal the decision [9]. When appealing a denied claim, be sure to call the insurance company to ask why it was denied. The reason for the denial may be something that you can correct and therefore get the decision reversed. For example, the insurance agent may tell you that they never received certain information from your doctor's office. By calling the doctor's office and having them send the requested information to the medical insurance company, you may get the denial reversed. It is not uncommon to have to appeal multiple times before a denied claim is reversed [9]. Please see Example 3, from this chapter, for further explanation.

Example 3. Medical Insurance: What To Know: Appealing a Denied Claim

Scenario: A 25-year-old woman went to her gynecologist for a routine pap smear. Without informing the patient, the doctor's office sent the patient's pap-smear specimen to a different laboratory than the laboratory the doctor's office had used for years. Consequently, the patient's specimen was processed and analyzed at the new laboratory. The patient received an $800 bill directly from the new laboratory. In the past, the patient did not receive a laboratory bill.

Discussion: The patient called her medical insurance company to ask why her pap-smear test results were not covered this year. It was then that the patient found out that the doctor's office has switched laboratories. Apparently, the new laboratory was not in network with the patient's insurance company. The medical insurance company told the patient to ask the doctor's office to put in writing that the doctor's office switched laboratories, unbeknownst to the patient. The patient obtained this letter from the doctor's office and sent it, along with a copy of the bill from the new laboratory, to her medical insurance company. With the received proof that the patient could not have known which laboratory her specimen was sent to, the medical insurance company waived their previous denial, and removed the charge for the patient. This example shows how spending the time to combat a denied claim could save you hundreds of dollars.

Summary: Medical Insurance: What To Know

- Having medical insurance can prevent bankruptcy and deep debt if there is a serious illness.
- As mandated in the Affordable Care Act, all Americans must have medical insurance. Americans without medical insurance will receive a tax penalty, with few exceptions.
- Medical insurance can be obtained from the government and/or private insurance companies.
- When appealing a denied claim, be sure to call the medical insurance company to ask why it was denied. They may tell you that they never received certain information from your doctor's office.

References

1. Why Should I have Health Insurance? Healthcare.gov. Retrieved 2014, April 4 from https://www.healthcare.gov/why-should-i-have-health-coverage/

2. ObamaCare Facts: Dispelling the Myths. Obama Care Explained. Retrieved 2014, April 8 from http://obamacarefacts.com/obamacare-explained.php

3. United States Census Bureau. CPS Health Insurance Definitions. Retrieved 2014, on April 8 from https://www.census.gov/hhes/www/hlthins/methodology/definitions/cps.html

4. US News and World Report. (Dec 16, 2013). Health: Health Insurance. Top insurance Companies. Heilbrunn, E. Retrieved 2014, April 8 from http://health.usnews.com/health-news/health-insurance/articles/2013/12/16/top-health-insurance-companies

5. United States Department of Labor. Health Plans and Benefits, Retrieved 2014, on April 8 from http://www.dol.gov/dol/topic/health-plans/

6. United States Department of Labor. Employees Benefit Security Administration. FAQs about COBRA Continuation Health Coverage. Retrieved 2014, April 8, from http://www.dol.gov/ebsa/faqs/faq-consumer-cobra.html

7. Merhar, C. Zane Benefits. (October 22, 2013). Employee Health Benefits and Insurance Blog: Pure Defined Contribution-A Health Insurance Allowance. Retrieved 2014, April 11 from http://www.zanebenefits.com/blog/bid/321718/Pure-Defined-Contribution-A-Health-Insurance-Allowance

8. Williams, JT. The Patient Advocate's Handbook: 300 Questions and Answers To Help You Care For Your Loved

One: At The Hospital And At Home. Panglossian Press: California.2010. pp 199-201.

9. Cohen, E. The Empowered Patient: How to Get the Right Diagnosis, Buy the Cheapest Drugs, Beat Your Insurance Company, and Get the Best Medical Care Every Time. Ballantine Books Trade Paperbacks: New York. 2010. p119.

7

Disability Insurance: What To Know

THIS CHAPTER IS FOCUSED MOSTLY ON private disability insurance as opposed to government programs. The information provided is for individuals who are truly disabled.

7.1 The Importance of Disability Insurance

An accident can occur at anytime, or an injury can develop slowly over time, leaving you unable to work. Therefore, it is critical to know what to do in order to maximize your chances of receiving the disability benefits you are entitled. If not for your own health, then for a loved one who has experienced a disabling event.

Individuals that become disabled while unemployed

If you become disabled while unemployed, you can apply for government aid via Social Security Disability Insurance or Supplemental Security Income, depending on your age and circumstance. Detailed information of the requirements for eligibility can be found at www.ssa.gov/disability

and www.ssa.gov/ssi. Additional information can be obtained at www.healthcare.gov.

Individuals that become disabled while employed
If, on the other hand, you become disabled while employed, you should first contact the private disability insurance program that your employer participates with and/or your private disability company.

When you are initially hired, this being before you are disabled, you should completely read and understand your disability contract supplied by your employer. When most people are hired, they are not disabled and therefore do not read the disability contract. As will be furthered explained in this chapter, this is a mistake that many individuals make. Before you are disabled, the best way to read your disability contract with understanding is to pretend that you are disabled while reading it. In this way, you will better comprehend the contract conditions.

A claimant is the person who is claiming to be disabled or injured. Some disability insurance companies will only cover a claimant who is unable to perform the tasks of his/her last job specifically, while others will cover the claimant who is unable to do any work. Such distinctions are critical because the claim can be denied simply based on the claimant's contract coverage, despite the claimant developing a disability that prevents the claimant from working his/her previous job.

7.2   The Motivation of Disability Insurance Companies
The disability insurance company is not a medical company. It is a business supported by investors with the idea that the

disability insurance company will generate money for them [1]. It is a "for profit" company and is therefore, designed to generate money, not spend money [2]. In short, the disability insurance company remains in good standing when it does not spend money. In this way, the company benefits when it is able to deny a claim.

As will be seen throughout this chapter, there are a variety of ways to deny a claim. Whistleblowers that have previously worked for a disability insurance company have stated that their co-workers, including claim adjusters and doctors, were rewarded if they met monthly claim denials [3].

Healthcare professionals that work for the disability insurance company may deny a claim without having all of the medical information [4]. Such an act would seem unreasonable for healthcare professionals, however their own jobs depend on denying claims. Because they are asked to review medical files in a limited, often short, time frame, it is possible that an incomplete medical file (for example, missing laboratory reports or radiographic images) is reviewed. Despite reviewing an incomplete file, healthcare professionals are required to render their medical opinion. Thus, your claim may be denied without a healthcare professional having a full account of your entire medical condition.

On the other hand, the disability insurance company cannot leave a claim open indefinitely. The company needs to render a decision about a claim after a designated amount of time. Otherwise, claimants could significantly delay the decision-making process by not having all of their documents submitted for review. If, for example, a claimant fails to submit a x-ray, the disability insurance company must still render a decision on what has been received. A denial in such case may be valid based on the limited documents received.

The monetary award received by a claimant ranges based on his/her contract with the disability insurance company. Usually, high-salaried individuals would receive a higher award. If you are a high-salaried individual filing for disability benefits, it benefits the insurer to deny your claim [5]. By denying a high-salaried individual an award, it can be equivalent to denying two or three lower-salaried individuals' award. Therefore, the disability insurance company would be compelled to deny such a claim and may choose to spend its own money, to justify such a decision. For example, the disability insurance company may hire a surveillance team to photograph and video the claimant in order to document his/her ability to work (1,6). Although the insurance company must pay the surveillance team, it is worth it for the company to pay the surveillance team as opposed to approving a claim from an individual who would unjustifiably receive disability benefits for years. The surveillance team will not capture the claimant performing duties that have been medically restricted, if the claimant is truly disabled. This is exemplified in Example 1 from this chapter.

The disability insurance company needs to protect its investors and integrity. It simply cannot provide disability benefits to every claimant blindly. By employing surveillance teams for example, the disability insurance company can verify if a claimant is truly disabled.

Example 1. Disability Insurance: What To Know: The Motivation of Disability Insurance Companies
<u>Scenario:</u> The claimant's salary had been over $300,000 per year. After being on disability for approximately five

months, the disability insurance company hired a two-man team to follow the claimant for three consecutive days. As the claimant stepped outside of his house, he received a phone call from an "unknown caller". Upon answering, the "unknown caller" hung up. The surveillance team began videotaping and photographing the claimant, as documented in the team's surveillance report. This suggests that the anonymous call was made to confirm the identity of the claimant.

Discussion: In this case, the insurance company did not succeed, as the disabled person was truly disabled and was surveyed performing the activities of a disabled person only.

The surveillance team charged the disability insurance company $5,000 for their efforts. For the disability insurance company, $5,000 is much less than the hundreds of thousands of dollars it would have to pay the claimant over the course of his disability.

7.3 Filing a Disability Claim

The case manager is an employee of the disability insurance company and is the first person assigned to your case and is often a non-medical professional. The case manager handles your claim by analyzing the validity of your claim. Your file may then be presented to healthcare professionals that work for the disability insurance company. They will also review your claim. Next, the case manager may suggest to his/her director that a surveillance team be used in your case. Unbeknownst to you (the claimant), a surveillance team is hired by the disability insurance company to record your behavior when away from a medical facility.

When you file for disability benefits, you will sign a waiver permitting the disability insurance company to have access to your full medical history, as it pertains to the claim. Therefore, your claim is composed of your medical history, past, present and future. When healthcare professionals review the claim, they analyze every component. This includes medications, number of medical professional visits, laboratory results, radiographic images, etc. An emphasis is placed on the restrictions listed by your treating doctor. Restrictions are what your treating doctor lists as activities that you are no longer able to do while disabled. These restrictions must specifically prevent you from working, in order for the claim not to be denied. Please see Example 2, in this chapter, for further clarification.

Example 2. Disability Insurance: What To Know: Filing a Claim

Medical Restriction
Scenario: A 52-year-old man, living in a rural setting, sustained a disabling injury. His doctor restricted him from lifting 50 lbs. and driving because of his new disability. He had been working as a tax account. Since his job did not require any lifting or driving, his claim was denied because he could still do his job. Although he needed to drive to get to work, the disability insurance company still denied his claim because their concern was not how he got to work, but rather that he could work.

Discussion: If a truck driver was restricted from driving by his treating doctor, then the disability insurance company will not be able to deny this claim so easily, as the truck driver's job is to drive.

The disability insurance company may attempt to disprove your treating doctor's restriction recommendation by stating that there is no medical evidence to warrant such a restriction. Often, this conclusion is reached by; the case manager, who does not have a medical degree; a nurse, who may or may not have experience with dealing with this condition; and/or a doctor, who has never examined the patient.

When the case manager or member of the disability insurance company's team is reviewing your medical file, normal findings will be highlighted. This is done in an attempt to justify that you can work. So, even if you have a disability, the company will highlight the medical reasons for you to be able to hold some type of job. If there is a medical abnormality, as demonstrated by laboratory or radiographic images, the case manager or member of the team, may ignore an abnormality, and focus on the normal findings discovered during the same exam. (Often times, a laboratory or radiographic test, will document both normal and abnormal findings. For example, when testing a patient's blood sample, the patient may be found to have diabetes, but also have a normal red blood cell count. A case manager or team member could ignore the diabetes finding and concentrate on the normal red blood count. This example is likely an exaggeration but is mentioned to simplify the concept of ignoring pertinent medical information. For a more realistic example, please refer to Example 3 in this chapter.)

Example 3. Disability Insurance: What To Know: Filing a Claim

Ignoring Medical Evidence
Scenario: A 55-year-old woman with relentless headaches and severe neck pain took a MRI. The MRI showed herniated ("slipped") discs in multiple locations in her neck. There were also some normal discs. The nurse working for the disability insurance company reviewed the MRI report and came to the conclusion that it was normal.

Discussion: To justify her conclusion, the nurse quoted sentences from the normal findings on the MRI, completely ignoring the gross, abnormal herniated discs. The claimant's claim was denied based on the nurse's assessment of a normal MRI.

If you are truly disabled, consider the following to reduce the chance of a claim denial:

- Read your employee disability contract before you develop a disability.
- Review the disability insurance company's disability form. You will receive this form after you make your claim.

- Ask your doctor to include evidence-based medical literature to support the answers on your disability insurance form.
- Remind your doctor of the importance for him/her to return calls from the disability insurance company.
- Follow your medical treatment plan. This includes attending medical visits and filling prescriptions.
- Comply with all questions made by the disability insurance company. Be completely honest and timely with their requests.

7.4 Waiting for the Disability Claim Decision

As a patient with a new disability, you may become overwhelmed from dealing with your sickness and from filling out paperwork for the disability insurance company. You will receive numerous phone calls, mail and emails from the disability insurance company. It is critical to know that all correspondence with the company is often recorded and reviewed, when assessing your claim. Even if your claim is approved, any correspondence with the disability insurance company will likely continue to be recorded, even months after your approval.

Filing for disability benefits is a long process. It will not serve you good fortune to be uncooperative with the case manager. There is no reason for you to give the case manager a personal reason to dislike you. The case manager is merely doing his/her job when reviewing your claim.

When reviewing your case, the disability insurance company analyzes your entire medical record. Your medication list, for example, could be targeted for further investigation. The disability insurance company will investigate the purpose of the medication, side effects and recommended doses for a particular condition.

The disability insurance company will ensure that you have attended your doctor visits and/or therapist treatments, as outlined by your treating doctor. The disability insurance company may decide to contact your treating doctor for further explanation of your condition. If the company is unable to reach your treating doctor for oral or written communication, your claim may be denied or you could lose your existing benefits. In this scenario, the company may deny your claim because your treating doctor has not returned your case manager's numerous phone calls or written inquiries. In order to avoid this, you may have to remind your doctor's office about filling out the claim requests from the disability insurance company.

Some of disability insurance companies may also require the names and addresses of all medical personnel you have seen, even if it is unrelated to your condition. So, if you are disabled due to a stroke, the disability insurance company may still require your medical notes from your last OB/GYN doctor visit. Keep in mind, that the disability insurance company can review **all** of your medical visits and prescriptions (with your permission). Example 4, in this chapter, highlights this concept.

Example 4. Disability Insurance: What To Know: Keeping a Claim Approved

Permission For The Disability Company To Review Any Medical Records

Scenario: A 20-year-old woman on disability due to a seizure disorder went to a gynecologist for a yeast infection. The disability company could request (with her permission) to have the medical records from the gynecologist office sent to them for review.

> Discussion: You should allow the disability insurance company all records that it requests because otherwise it may seem that you are attempting to hide something from them that is relevant to your claim.

The disability insurance company may require that you apply for Social Security Disability Insurance. Acceptance into that program will offset a portion of the benefits the disability insurance company must provide you. If you are found eligible for Social Security Disability benefits, the amount awarded to you from the government will be deducted from the disability insurance company's award. In this way, the disability insurance company will pay less from its bank, but your overall award could remain the same since the government subsidizes some of it. A claimant approved for Social Security Disability Insurance also receives government-issued health insurance, Medicare.

7.5 Keeping Your Claim Approved
Once you begin receiving disability benefits, you will be sent numerous documents to complete. Depending on the case manager, they may want monthly contact with you regarding your condition and your daily activities of living. This allows them to stay up-to-date on your situation. The case manager will look to see if you are attending your medical visits, they will review your current medications and they will check to see if anything has changed that would allow for you to work.

Depending on the disability insurance company and your condition, each month, you may be sent forms from the disability insurance company requesting any current changes in your condition, including the names of doctors seen, therapy sessions attended and medical tests performed. This information is used every month, along with any medical notes from your treating doctor's office, to assess your medical progress. The disability form may also request the name of any medical professional seen, regardless of the relevance to your disability claim.

If you opt not to allow the disability insurance company access to all of your medical records, this may provide cause for the company to believe that you are hiding medical information from them. There is no reason to raise such suspicion, so it is best to release your medical notes, regardless of their relevance to your disability claim.

The case manager will review your medication list. First, there is an analysis to see if the medication ordered is appropriate for the alleged disability. Second, the side effects of the drugs are examined. For example, if a particular drug is known to make a patient drowsy, and the patient is taking this medication in the morning or mid-day, it would make it difficult for the patient to work during normal business hours.

7.5.1 The Independent Medical Examination (IME)

Eventually, you may receive an invitation from the disability insurance company to see a doctor of the company's choosing. You will be asked to see the chosen doctor for an independent medical examination (IME). The disability insurance company chooses a doctor from their list of doctors who have agreed to conduct examinations on claimants. These doctors receive substantial fees from the disability insurance company. Some doctors dedicate much of their week to conducting multiple independent medical examinations, as working with the disability insurance company can be profitable.

Given that these medical providers are on the disability insurance company's payroll, like the case manager, the medical provider may have an incentive to find a claimant not disabled [7]. After all, if a medical provider documents that "too many" of the claimants are in fact disabled, the disability insurance company may be prompted to find a different medical provider who yields results that benefit the company financially [7]. Thus, if a medical provider wants to keep the lucrative side business of performing independent medical examinations, he/she has an incentive to produce results that are favorable to the disability insurance company's for-profit model [7]. In this way, the insurer has its own doctors to oppose your claim [1].

This is not to say that independent medical examiners are "for hire" and that they will dismiss their own medical opinion for the sake of meeting a disability insurance company's preference for denied claims. In fact, independent medical examiners should comply with the guidelines set for this type of medical evaluation as stipulated by federal, local, state and medical society guidelines [8]. In this setting, the independent medical examiner should provide his/her genuine medical opinion without the influence of insurers.

Yet, in the setting of an independent medical examination, the claimant is viewed more as a claimant than as a patient. For example, the independent medical examiner may be informed of the amount of benefit money the claimant receives from the disability company. This should not be relevant when analyzing a patient's medical condition.

Other evidence that the claimant is viewed more as a claimant than as a patient, is the following: the disability insurance company chooses the medical provider, sets up the appointment, sends the claimant's medical chart to the medical provider, pays for the appointment and receives the report of the visit directly from the medical provider. Additionally, the claimant is often not given the medical provider's opinion about his/her condition or a recommendation of possible treatment options for him/her. In fact, independent medical examiners may be encouraged to inform the patient that the scope of the IME cannot substitute for a standard physician examination [9]. And that care should be sought elsewhere [9]. The claimant is usually not given a copy of the medical provider's report.

The independent medical examiner may determine that you are not disabled, even though your personal doctor determined that you are disabled. The case manager can then opt to favor the opinion of the independent medical examiner, and can subsequently deny your claim.

You should attend the independent medical examination with a companion. Answer the questions asked by the medical provider, and nothing more. Finally, be pleasant and cooperative. This will reduce your stress and keep the visit as positive as possible.

7.6 Appealing a Denied Claim

The approach you take to reverse your denied disability claim depends on whether you possessed personal disability insurance or group disability insurance before you became sick. *Group disability insurance* is offered by your company and covers all eligible employees. *Personal disability insurance,* on the other hand, is paid directly by a private disability insurance company generally after you meet with a representative from that company.

7.6.1 Group Disability Insurance Protocol for Appeals

If you have group insurance and your claim is denied, you can appeal this decision directly to the disability insurance company. Of course, if this company denied you once, this could happen again. Being denied disability benefits can result in both income and health insurance loss for you. This depends on how the contract between your employer and the disability insurance company is stated.

When your claim is denied, you will receive a denial letter from the disability insurance company. Once your disability insurance carrier has denied your claim, it is difficult to have the decision reversed. A letter will be sent to you, furnished by the disability insurance company, stating the company's regret and reasons for not being able to grant you disability benefits.

You must write an appeal by addressing every reason listed for the denial in the denial letter. An explanation, with evidence, must be provided in response to each issue raised in the denial letter. Despite you being sick and stressed from losing income and possibly health insurance, you are left with the responsibility of collecting supportive evidence of your disability. Evidence comes in the form of clear medical abnormalities indicated in your medical file, that were "overlooked", by the case manager. (See Example 3, from this chapter).

Other evidence which you could submit when appealing a denial, is a letter written by your treating doctor. You can ask your doctor to write a letter to the disability insurance company justifying your disability. The disability insurance company may still deny the claim, despite your treating doctor's recommendation. Additionally, the insurance company's team may not include a specialist or could include a medical professional with less expertise than your own treating physician [10].

Once the appeal including all evidence gathered is submitted, the disability insurance company can take months to render an opinion on the appeal and in the meantime, you are denied benefits. The company may reject the appeal and uphold the decision to deny your claim, again. At this point, the claimant can submit a second appeal. If denied again, there may be opportunity for another appeal.

7.6.2 Private Disability Insurance Protocol for Appeals

Individuals with personal health insurance usually do not go through the process of writing appeals to the company that denied them. Instead, individuals with personal health insurance can go directly to court and fight the denial of disability benefits.

7.6.3 What You Can Do if Your Disability Insurance Claim Has Been Denied

You may want to hire a lawyer if your claim is denied. Some law firms boast successful appeal rates. Keep in mind, these lawyers are paid by you, so you will either have to pay them out of your own pocket or they will share in the successful appeal awards. Lawyers, such as these, can be found online by searching "disability insurance lawyers".

If you decide not to hire a lawyer and appeal your denied claim yourself, you may want to do the following: request a copy of your entire claim file, including all documentation of every conversation, email and medical notes from the disability insurance company. If complete, it should contain all intra-office discussions regarding your case made by your case manager, medical director, nurses and doctors. There may be no charge to you for the disability insurance company to send you a copy of your complete file. Reviewing these notes, may give you a better insight as to why your case was denied.

Summary: Disability Insurance: What To Know
- While waiting for your disability benefits, cooperate with the disability insurance company's case manager.
- What you can do to keep your disability benefits
  - Maintain strict compliance with medical recommendations, including filling prescriptions and attending all medical appointments.
  - Submit ongoing medical documents when requested.
  - Cooperate and attend the independent medical examination (IME). Consider this as an appointment that <u>cannot</u> be missed. If possible, bring a companion with you.
- How to appeal a denied claim with <u>Group Disability Insurance</u>
  - Obtain a lawyer or represent yourself
  - Submit Evidence For Appeal
  - Use existing documentation (such as laboratory and radiographic data) that may have been overlooked
  - Ask your treating doctor to write a letter explaining why you are disabled.
  - Request a copy of your file from the disability insurance company.
- How to appeal a denied claim with <u>Personal Disability Insurance</u>
  1. Obtain a lawyer or represent yourself
  2. Request a copy of your file from the disability insurance company.

References

1. Elkind & Shea. Top Ten Reasons How An Insurer Takes Advantage of You. Retrieved May 2013, from http://www.disabilitybenefitslawfirm.com/articles_TopTen.htm
2. Whitehead and Associates, LLP. (2010). Long Term Disability. Retrieved May 2013, from http://www.disabilitydenials.com/long-term-disability.html.
3. Pierce, S. (2012, August). Unum Lawsuit Filed by Disabled Woman Denied Disability Insurance Benefits. Top Drug Lawsuits.
4. Sokolove Law, LLC. (2003-13). Tips for Filing A Long Term Disability Appeal. Retrieved in May 2013, from http://www.sokolovelaw.com/legal-help/disability-insurance-lawyer/long-term-disability-denial/insurance-bad-faith/filing-tips.
5. Goselin, P. Attorneys Dell and Schaefer. A Classic Unum Provident Denial. Retrieved in May 2013, from http://www.diattorney.com/a-classic-unum-provident-denial/.
6. Comitz/Beethe (2012). Misuse of Surveillance in Investigation of Disability Insurance Claims. Retrieved in May 2013, from http://www.disabilitycounsel.net/Surveillance.html
7. Spencer, R.F. (2010). Are Independent Medical Examiners Truly Independent? *Pain Physician*, Jan-Feb;13(1):92-3; author reply 93-4.
8. Ky P., Hameed, H., & Christo P.J. (2009). Independent Medical Examinations: Facts and Fallacies. *Pain Physician*, Sep-Oct;12(5):811-8.
9. Baum K. (2005). Independent Medical Examinations: An Expanding Source of Physician Liability. *Ann Intern Med 2005*, (21), 974-978.

10. J.Bemis, Roach & Reed. (2013). Department of Labor Rules Governing ERISA. Retrieved May 2013 from http://www.brrlaw.com/practice-areas/long-term-disability/erisa/.

8

Medical Fraud And Medical Malpractice

MEDICAL FRAUD AND MALPRACTICE ARE VERY rare; you are unlikely to encounter them. If your condition worsens, it does not mean that the doctor was incompetent. Medical fraud is defined as hiding or misrepresenting the medical standard for a financial gain [1]. Medical malpractice is harming a patient after conducting substandard medical care. Both practices involve medical "professionals" that rely on your trust in them to treat you in a medically correct manner.

8.1 Identifying Medical Fraud

Medical fraud is when a medical professional knowingly hides or misrepresents the medical standard for a financial gain [1]. Medical abuse is the same as medical fraud but is usually done unknowingly by the medical professional [1].

There must be "clear and convincing" evidence of fraud, malice, and/or gross negligence to prove the accusation [2]. Some of the most common types of fraud and abuse are misrepresentation of billing for services not rendered; altering claim forms for higher payments; falsification of information in medical record documents; billing for services that were not performed or misrepresenting the types of services that were provided; billing for supplies not provided; and providing medical services that are unnecessary based on the patient's "condition" [1]. (Please see Example 1, from this chapter, to exemplify the latter.) Other examples of potential medical fraud/abuse is when a healthcare provider promises patients "miracle cures" or accepts fees from patients while using mystical or spiritual powers [3].

Example 1. Medical Fraud And Medical Malpractice: Identifying Medical Fraud
Scenario: A 16-year-old female patient had an x-ray of her mouth as her dentist felt she had another cavity. On the x-ray, the dentist pointed out the tooth in need of a cavity filling. After two years of seeing the same dentist and the dentist stating that the girl had a cavity at each visit, the girl's mother requested a copy of the x-ray and took it to another dentist for a second opinion. The second dentist saw no indication or need for a cavity filling.

Discussion: The 16-year-old patient had seen the same dentist for the last 2 years, twice each year. Prior to this, she had never had a cavity. The current dentist claimed that she had at least one cavity at each visit. In total, he had given her 5 fillings and had billed her family accordingly. For whatever reason, he took an x-ray of the patient's mouth this time. Luckily for the patient, this documentation saved her from additional unnecessary dental procedures. In this scenario, there may or may not have been medical fraud. Because she had never had an x-ray before, she could not prove if the previous 5 fillings were warranted or not.

Billing fraud can happen in a variety of ways. For example, a fraudulent doctor may "inflate" a patient's diagnosis so that he/she can bill the insurance company for treating a more costly disease. In this way, the doctor will receive re-imbursement for treating a condition that the insurance company has labeled as deserving a higher reimbursement, even though the he/she actually treated for a different, less reimbursable disease. This could have effects on the un-knowing patient, as his/her insurance company would cite a more complicated condition than what the patient actu-ally has. Additionally, the patient may feel that he/she has a more complicated condition if he/she were somehow able to review and understand the billing codes.

Fraud can also be accomplished by the medical profes-sional that will not pay to update his/her medical equip-ment. Consequently, patients may be treated with machines and other instruments that are outdated.

Some medical professionals may choose to blame others for their own error. That is, a doctor may try to convince a pa-tient that another doctor caused the problem, when in reality the problem was caused by the current doctor. Therefore, if a patient intends to report medical fraud, it is important to iden-tify the appropriate doctor. A conniving doctor is relying on your lack of medical education as a means to prevent you from realizing that he/she actually caused your problem. (Please see Example 4, in this chapter, for further clarification.)

8.2 Identifying Medical Malpractice

"Negligence becomes medical malpractice, and the basis of a medical malpractice lawsuit, when it results in undue injury to a patient" [4]. Therefore, medical malpractice is the act of harming a patient after conducting negligent, substandard medical care. Victims of malpractice must document that they relied on the medical providers advice and/or treatment that directly resulted in the victim's harm.

If you feel that a medical professional has engaged in medical malpractice, you must analyze your situation. For example, if a patient dies from a particular disease, the doctor may not have been negligent, despite the fact that another doctor would have treated the patient differently. This is because there are legal criteria that must be proven to establish any claim of medical negligence. The following are the criteria as stated by "The American Medical Association (AMA)...[for]... negligence" [3]:

1. "Duty. Patients must show that a [patient-physician] relationship existed in which the physician owed the patient a duty" [3].
2. "Derelict. Patients must show that the physician failed to comply with the standards of the profession" [3]. "The patient must also prove that he or she sustained an injury that would not have occurred in the absence of this negligence. In other words, the patient must prove that the negligence caused the injury" [5]. "An unfavorable outcome by itself is not malpractice" [5].
3. "Direct cause. Patients must show that any damages were a direct cause of a physician's breach of duty" [3].
4. "Damages. Patients must prove that they suffered injury" [3].

Duty, the first criteria, refers to "the patient-physician relationship". This is an established relationship between you and your physician in which you expect medically sound advisement regarding your condition [6]. It is your doctor's duty to offer you sound medical advice. Such a relationship is usually established in the office but can alternatively be established in a non-medical environment, such as on a golf course.

Regardless of the location, when you seek advice from a doctor, the patient-physician relationship is established and it is that doctor's duty, or responsibility, to offer you sound medical advice. If a doctor makes a recommendation to a person, even a friend, then the patient-physician relationship has been established. Thus, regardless of the formality of the environment, if a person obtains medical advice from a doctor, then the patient-physician relationship has been formed. This is exemplified in Example 2 in this chapter.

Example 2. Medical Fraud And Medical Malpractice: Identifying Medical Malpractice

Duty Criteria
Scenario: A father and son-in-law went fishing one weekend. While there, the father asked his son-in-law to look at an irregular mole on his cheek. The son-in-law was a well-known dermatologist. The son-in-law told his father-in-law that the lesion was completely benign and to not think of it again. Two years later, the father presented to the emergency room confused and disoriented. It was determined that he had metastatic melanoma to the brain. The father had

never had the original mole on his cheek examined since his son-in-law had looked at it while fishing years earlier.

Discussion: In such a scenario, the court may find that the father followed the recommendation of his son-in-law based on the son-in-law being a doctor, not a relative. Therefore, a patient-physician relationship was established. The son-in-law, therefore, could be liable for his recommendation.

Derelict, the second criteria, offers room for interpretation. It involves establishing the standard of care. Determining the standard of care is based on the medical practices in a given locale, not necessarily the cutting edge technology from abroad or a large academic setting in the United States. Thus, if you are treated with a particular medication, with detrimental results and it is determined that there was a better "drug available", your doctor may not have been negligent. That is, if other similarly situated doctors (meaning other doctors in that environment with similar training background and academic exposure) would have treated you the same way as your doctor did, then the care you received was not legally substandard. There are many ways to explore and manipulate this conclusion. For example, a lawyer could investigate if the doctor should have taken recent medical education courses to increase his/her awareness of medical advancements. Thus, there can be many ways to claim if an action was standard or substandard. This is exemplified in Example 3 in this chapter.

Example 3. Medical Fraud And Medical Malpractice: Identifying Medical Malpractice

Derelict Criteria

Scenario: A teenage boy was seen by his family doctor in a small, rural town upon breaking his wrist while playing baseball. The doctor reset the bone, placed his arm in a cast and prescribed pain medication. A few weeks later, it was determined that the bone was not set correctly and the boy would need to have surgery.

Discussion: It is possible that the family practitioner would not be at fault as he may have set the bone to the best of his ability and that the other physicians in this town would have treated the patient in a similar manner. Also, without access to x-rays and other radiographic images, this physician may have not performed below the standard of care in that region of the country. Had the boy's accident occurred in a town where medical testing and tools were abundant, the doctor may be at fault for setting a bone incorrectly if it led to further damage.

Direct cause, the third criteria, states that the doctor caused the patient harm. Obviously, if you are claiming malpractice, you must make the claim against the person that actually caused your harm. Example 4 demonstrates how in one medical malpractice case, an innocent doctor and others were blamed for harming a patient.

Example 4. Medical Fraud And Medical Malpractice: Identifying Medical Malpractice

Direct Cause Criteria

<u>Scenario:</u> After having a skin cancer removed, by a surgeon, a patient felt that the scar on her cheek was too large. When she informed the surgeon of her disappointment with the result, the unscrupulous surgeon told her that it was her previous doctor's fault. Therefore, she decided to sue her former dermatologist, as well as the dermatologist's entire staff and the laboratory that had correctly diagnosed her cancer. Her husband cited that he could not look at his wife due to the scar; so he also sued those mentioned above.

<u>Discussion:</u> Ultimately, the suit was dropped by the presiding judge as all of the individuals who were being sued, did not cause the scar on her face. Instead, it was her surgeon who had left a large scar behind. (Incidentally, the size of her scar was reflective of the size of her cancer, and therefore, the surgeon's work may have very well been within the standard of care, so he too would likely not have been successfully sued against.)

Patients sometimes do not understand what is meant by the fourth criteria, damages. The simplest way to think of damages is to consider them as a measurement of the patient's loss. In this way, the damages could range from minimal to devastating, based on the legal value placed on the loss. This is exemplified in Example 5 in this chapter.

> ## Example 5. Medical Fraud and Medical Malpractice: Identifying Medical Malpractice
>
> *Damages Criteria*
> <u>Scenario:</u> A patient's normal right foot was mistakenly removed during surgery, as opposed to the diseased left foot.
>
> <u>Discussion:</u> In this scenario, it is undeniable that the patient suffered an irreversible detrimental loss. This type of damage is clear and would likely lead to a settlement offer for the patient.

All four criteria (duty, derelict, direct cause and damages) must be met for a claim of negligence/medical malpractice to legally have merit.

Examples of Medical Malpractice

Medical malpractice can take many forms. Here are some examples that might lead to a lawsuit:

- "Failure to diagnose or misdiagnosis
- Misreading or ignoring laboratory results
- Unnecessary surgery
- Surgical errors or wrong site surgery
- Improper medication or dosage
- Poor follow-up or aftercare
- Premature discharge
- Disregarding or not taking appropriate patient history
- Failure to order proper testing
- Failure to recognize symptoms" [5]

If a doctor/nurse feels that a particular case could lead to a malpractice suit, he/she may unscrupulously opt to remove or alter damaging information from a chart, if he/she feels that a mistake was made. If such action is discovered, this doctor/nurse will likely lose the case if it goes to trial. As a patient, you can protect yourself by requesting a copy of your medical note, after each visit, if you have a complicated condition. As stated in Chapter 4.2.1, During The Medical Visit: Medical Documentation of Your Condition: The Medical (SOAP) Note, a new medical (SOAP) note is written to document your visit at each visit. Having copies of your medical notes could provide proof in the future if there is an accusation that your notes had been subsequently altered or removed.

8.3   Reporting Medical Fraud

Medical fraud is a component of what is called healthcare fraud [7]. Reporting healthcare fraud is central to the well being of the greater community [8]. Patients and medical providers must be committed to address abuse issues and take a moral and ethical stand against fraud in the healthcare environment [1]. Healthcare fraud costs the United States approximately $80 billion a year [8].

Patients and healthcare professionals can report their concerns of medical fraud by contacting the healthcare professional's medical licensing board. Reporting a healthcare professional to the appropriate licensing board is a power that both patients and other healthcare professionals have. In fact, if a healthcare professional suspects fraud, he/she is ethically obligated to report it. In this way, healthcare workers should report if another healthcare provider is deceiving a patient.

Like healthcare professionals, it is important for a patient to report fraudulent medical behavior. There is a specific medical licensing board for each of the varied healthcare professionals. You can access medical licensing boards by searching the Internet. For example, if you wanted to report a neurologist, search the Internet with key phrases like, "reporting medical fraud to neurology medical licensing board".

Depending on the specific specialty of a doctor, he/she may be a member of multiple medical boards. In such a case, the patient should report the fraudulent doctor to all medical boards that the doctor is affiliated with. Please see Example 6, in this chapter, for further demonstration.

Example 6. Medical Fraud And Medical Malpractice: Reporting Medical Fraud

Scenario: A patient became highly suspicious of his internist's billing practices. When making a call to his internist, he was placed on hold and learned from the voice recording that his doctor was board certified by both the American Board of Pediatrics and the American Board of Internal Medicine.

Discussion: If he decided to report such a doctor for suspected fraud, he would contact both the American Board of Pediatrics and the American Board of Internal Medicine.

What if the doctor that is suspected of fraud was never board certified?

If your doctor is not board certified, you should report the fraudulent behavior to your state governmental agency against medical fraud. (Even if your doctor is board certified, you could also report him/her to your state governmental agency against medical fraud.) The state has the power to revoke a general medical license from a doctor for good cause. If revoked, the doctor will lose the right to practice medicine. To locate your state governmental agency against medical fraud search the Internet. Use key words and phrases like "state governmental agency department of health against medical fraud". For example, if you wanted to report a gynecologist in Nebraska, search the Internet with key words and phrases like, "Nebraska Department of Health reporting medical fraud".

Are there any other places to report medical fraud?
Many medical professionals are often members of various medical societies. A patient with a real concern should contact a medical society for additional guidance.

You may be able to find out which societies or associations the physician may belong to by requesting guidance from the medical licensing board. Some doctors' offices list the doctor's societal membership in a voice recording when a patient is placed on hold. If this is not helpful, then one must investigate by conducting Internet searches. Medical societies can be found by searching the Internet. For example, if you wanted to report a pathologist in Louisiana to a medical society, search the Internet with key phrases to find the society, such as "Louisiana pathology medical society".

8.4 Launching a Medical Malpractice Lawsuit
If you sustained injury by a healthcare provider, you may consider launching a medical malpractice lawsuit. Before doing so, you must realize that certain criteria must be met in the eyes of the court to consider the merit of your claim. These

criteria are duty, derelict, direct cause and damage [3]. (These criteria are explained in detail earlier in this chapter, in Section 8.2, Identifying Medical Malpractice.)

After you have satisfactorily established that these criteria have been met in your case, you will need to find a malpractice attorney. You may have to contact many before you find the one that will take your case. While an attorney speaks with you, he/she is evaluating the merits of your claim. He/she is deciding whether your claims fulfill the criteria from a legal standard, not from your perspective. Because some malpractice attorneys must pay for the case out of his/her own pocket, including paying the high costs for consultants such as expert witnesses, an attorney often will not take on a malpractice case unless he/she truly believes that he/she will win. Otherwise, the attorney loses tens of thousands of dollars for every malpractice case they take on, but do not win.

When launching a medical malpractice lawsuit, an attorney will look through your medical records and investigate any healthcare professional that you may have encountered, as being party to your injury. In other words, when filing a case on your behalf, the attorney will investigate your primary provider as well as ancillary staff. This means that nurses, laboratories, doctors and companies may be "named" (accused of malpractice) in addition to your primary doctor. However, be sure that the healthcare professional that caused your problem is the one named in the malpractice lawsuit. Example 4, from this chapter, reiterates this point. Be sure to launch a malpractice claim against the actual culprit of your case and avoid making claims against the wrong healthcare provider.

Naming an innocent person in a medical malpractice case can cause significant damage to that person. Doctors, for example, that are named in malpractice lawsuits must report each incident to their licensing boards and their insurance companies. Regardless if the malpractice case goes to trial or not, the doctor will carry this accusation with him for the rest of his life. Therefore, before commencing in a medical malpractice lawsuit, it is best to be sure of the merits of your claims. Example 7, from this chapter, shows the deadly result of an ancillary healthcare professional accused of medical malpractice.

Example 7. Medical Fraud And Medical Malpractice: Launching a Medical Malpractice Lawsuit

Scenario: A 25-year-old female doctor that had recently graduated from medical school visited patients with her instructor, in a hospital. Because she had just graduated from medical school, it was the hospital's policy that new doctors follow a more experienced doctor for the first few months. The 25-year-old doctor was basically an apprentice of the experienced doctor. She did not treat the patients directly, but her name was included in every medical note, along with the experienced doctor. The experienced doctor made all decisions regarding the patients.

Discussion: One of the patients seen by these two medical professionals suffered from an alleged incident of medical malpractice. The patient hired an attorney who reviewed all of the medical notes. The attorney saw that the 25-year-old doctor's name was on some of the medical notes. Ultimately, both the experienced doctor and the young doctor were formally accused of medical malpractice. When the young doctor learned that she was being sued, she was devastated. Her career had not yet begun and she had been accused of harming a patient. Although she had not directly treated the patient, she would always have to explain why she was named in such a case and would also have to stand trial. For these reasons and because news of alleged malpractice spreads through out the medical community, she committed suicide.

Summary: Medical Fraud And Medical Malpractice
- Suspected cases of medical fraud can be reported to state medical licensing boards, specialty certifying boards and/or specialty medical societies.
- You will likely need a medical malpractice lawyer to launch a successful medical malpractice lawsuit.
- Accusations of medical fraud and medical malpractice should have merit. Such an accusation made against an innocent healthcare provider could destroy his/her career.

References

1. William J Rudman, W.J., Eberhardt, J.S., Pierce, W. & Hart-Hester, S. (2009, Sept 16). Healthcare Fraud and Abuse. *Perspect Health Inf Manag.* 2009; 6(Fall): 1g.

2. Thornton, R.G. (2006). Malice/Gross Negligence. *Proc (Bayl Univ Med Cent).* 2006 October; 19(4): 417–418.

3. Booth, K.A., Whicker, L.G., Wyman, T.D., Pugh, D.J. & Thompson, S. Legal and Ethical Issues in Medical Practice, Including HIPAA. *Medical Assisting: Administrative and Clinical Procedures.* (pp. 38-45). McGraw-Hill.

4. McCarthy, J.S. *Medical Malpractice vs Medical Negligence.* Avvo: Have no Legal Fear. Retrieved in June 2013, from http://www.avvo.com/legal-guides/ugc/ medical-malpractice-vs-medical-negligence

5. American Board of Professional Liability Attorneys. What is Medical Malpractice?. Retrieved in June 2013, from http://www.abpla.org/what-is-malpractice.

6. Ratushny, V. & Allen, H. The Effects of Medical Malpractice on Dermatology and Related Specialities. Journal of Medical Science Research. Sept 30, 2007. 1(1)

7. Health Care Fraud. (March 2013). In *Wikipedia.* Retrieved 2013, June 7, from http://en.wikipedia.org/wiki/ Health_care_fraud

8. The Federal Bureau of Investigation. *Health Care Fraud.* Retrieved 2013, June 7, from http://www.fbi.gov/ about-us/investigate/white_collar/health-care-fraud

9

Trends In Healthcare

HEALTHCARE DEVELOPMENTS ARE REVIEWED IN THIS chapter. The topics chosen offer a new approach to longstanding issues in medicine and are simply fascinating. With the implementation of technology and policy changes, the future of healthcare in the U.S. is promising and exciting!

9.1 E-Health

E-health is the use of electronic technology (such as the internet and/or cellphone technology) to improve healthcare. The benefits of e-Health have already revolutionized healthcare and new benefits will emerge as technology develops further. The application of e-Health is extensive, as it can be used in almost every facet of healthcare. At this time, e-Health is most popularly applied in social media arenas, electronic medical records (EMR), electronic health records (EHR), administrative processing, telemedicine, and patient compliance. Thus, there are many areas of medicine that are affected by e-Health.

One such area is the transferring of health related issues, including your medical record and general public health information, to various parties. These parties can include patients, doctors, insurance companies and the government. E-Health provides a new medium for interaction and collaboration among institutions, healthcare professionals, healthcare providers and the public [1]. According to the Open Clinical website, e-Health can accomplish this by:

- "Supporting the delivery of care tailored to individual patients;
- Improving transparency and accountability of care processes and facilitating shared care across boundaries;
- Aiding evidence-based practice and error reduction;
- Improving diagnostic accuracy and treatment appropriateness;
- Improving access to effective healthcare by reducing barriers created, for example, by physical location or disability;
- Facilitating patient empowerment for self-care and health decision making;
- Improving cost-efficiency by streamlining processes, reducing waiting times and waste." [2]

Such improvements include quality, cost-efficiency and access to healthcare [2]. Multiple parties benefit from e-Health simultaneously. In other words, it does not benefit insurance companies without benefiting patients at the same time.

Because e-Health simply refers to electronic use in the healthcare system, it includes many more uses than what has been mentioned above. It is also includes virtual reality, robotics, multi-media (e.g. CD-ROM), digital imaging, computer assisted surgery, wearable and portable monitoring systems, and health portals [2]. E-Health is used by health systems management facilities for commerce and business practices [1].

9.1.1 Patient and Administrative Office Benefits

Electronic Medical Records (EMR)
Technology will continue to improve doctor office visits. By digitizing your information, the doctor, staff and insurance companies can more easily and quickly transfer data. The first step in the digitizing of your information is done in the form of an electronic medical record (EMR).

The electronic medical record (EMR) is a digital version of a patient's chart [3]. (The chart includes all of the information that was discussed in Chapter 4.2.1, During The Medical Visit: Medical Documentation of Your Condition: The Medical (SOAP) Note.) The EMR is an account of a patient's chart at that one specific doctor's office [3].

Electronic Health Record (EHR)
The electronic health record (EHR), on the other hand, includes all of the information found in the EMR and shares it with other healthcare professionals [3]. Thus, unlike the EMR, the EHR includes all of the information in the EMR plus all of the information from the patient's other doctor visits. Thus, EHR can be shared between separate doctors' offices, while EMR remains at one office.

"EHRs are designed to reach out beyond the health organization that originally collects and compiles the information. They are built to share information with other health care providers, such as laboratories and specialists, so they contain information from all the clinicians involved in the patient's care. The information moves with the patient—to the specialist, the hospital, the nursing home, the next state or even across the country. EHRs are designed to be accessed by all people involved in the [patient's] care—*including the patients themselves*" [3].

Potentially, with EHRs, all members of the team have ready access to the latest information allowing for more co-ordinated, patient-centered care [3]. For example:

- "The information gathered by the primary care provider tells the emergency department clinician about the patient's life threatening allergy, so that care can be adjusted appropriately, even if the patient is unconscious" [3].
- "A patient can log on to his own record and see the trend of the lab results over the last year, which can help motivate him to take his medications and keep up with the lifestyle changes that have improved the numbers" [3].
- "The lab results run last week are already in the record to tell the specialist what she needs to know without running duplicate tests" [3].

The administrative office staff of a doctor's office benefits greatly with the use of EHR as it helps to coordinate the patient's chart and the flow of information to other healthcare professionals. Cumbersome duties once performed by staff members are now more quickly and reliably done electronically. For example, booking appointments, saving patient information, and updating billing information can now be done electronically. Additionally, because doctors can electronically order prescriptions, the administrative office staff receives fewer phone calls from pharmacies and patients regarding prescriptions. Some doctor's offices allow you to fill in your health information and insurance forms electronically, prior to you visit, which potentially reduces your wait time in the office. If done without error, the overall improved efficiency of the administrative office staff is likely immeasurable due to EHR. The very application of EHR is designed to reduce errors.

Personal Health Record (PHR)

Personal health records (PHR) are the patient's electronic health record (EHR) but the patient has access to it. The patient adds information he/she chooses to include in it. The patient also decides who has access to these records. However, be careful, as these "personal" notes may be retrieved for legal purposes at a later time.

There are a host of PHR programs for you to enter your health data. PHR programs may be provided by employers and insurance companies. You can also decide to access such a program on your own by doing an Internet search for "PHR health records". The benefit of you entering your health information keeps you on top of every aspect of your overall health.

Patients can access medication information from multiple providers, reconcile them, update them, and share them with their physician using PHR technology [4]. "A patient-initiated medication reconciliation system is likely to be more accurate, as patients know not only what has been prescribed but what they are actually taking… advanced PHRs provide decision support tools, such as checking for drug allergies… and allowing patients to anticipate potential medication errors and alert physicians to them" [4].

Internet Applications

There are websites that patients and/or doctors can use to benefit the doctor's administrative office. These innovative websites offer solutions to finding a doctor, appointment scheduling, filling out forms, entering data into the electronic health record (EHR) and sharing this information with other healthcare professionals. Obviously, these benefits also help the patient and the doctor.

There are also websites that offer health information. These websites should not be used in place of pamphlets supplied by your doctor's offices. If you find a website that relays health information, be sure to read articles that have been written by healthcare professionals, and not amateurs. Governmental health sites, such as the United States Department of Health and Human Services (www.hhs.gov) are a trusted source for such information. Regardless of where you obtain health-related information, be sure to review it with your doctor.

Mobile Applications

There is an application that can give your doctor access to medical records, medication lists, and e-prescribing functionality [7]. "This allows the clinician in any location to manage the patient's medication renewals and review the patient's medical records, thereby enabling the clinician to respond to the patient's requests for refills at any time" [7].

Medication Adherence Solutions

Compliance refers to a patient taking their medication as directed. If you follow the prescribed regimen, you are considered "compliant". If, on the other hand, you do not follow the recommended regimen, then you are "non-compliant" or "not completely compliant". The destructive result of non-compliance is exemplified in Example 2 from Chapter 5.1.2, After The Medical Visit: Do You Understand Treatment Recommendations?.

A patient's compliance, or adherence, to a medication regimen can have a direct effect on treatment success, especially in patients with chronic diseases. Poor adherence with prescribed therapy often results in decreased efficacy, which is problematic for patients and physicians and adds extensive costs to the healthcare system, as the patient may not improve [8]. However, E-Health offers potential solutions to the lack of patient compliance/adherence to a medical regimen. Some solutions require Internet access while other use mobile technology.

The Internet can provide interactive and responsive programs in the healthcare arena [9,10]. It can serve as a powerful resource to remind you to follow your prescribed medical regimen as directed. Such use could get you more involved in your healthcare. This could be accomplished by offering individualized attention via messages, the incorporation of interactive and continued self-monitoring, feedback, and information exchange [10].

Although there are a number of homecare devices available to remind you to take your medication, such as a vibrating watch alarm, there are newer devices that are Internet based [7]. The Internet based devices document if and when pills are removed from a pillbox, for example [7]. The documentation is typically transmitted via computer over the Internet; this type of reporting service is called *tele-homecare [7].*

For example, there is a device that documents each time a single pill is removed from a pillbox [7]. Another device has a microchip linked to the cap that sounds an alert when it is time to take the medication [7]. " When the cap is opened, the chip will date- and time-stamp the opening and closing of the container. At any time, the chip can send a radio signal to a reader that records the stored events on a Windows-based computer. The computer can transfer the adherence monitoring data over the Internet to the patient's health care team [7]." There is another device that will send a prearranged reminder message to the patient, if the medication is not removed from the device within a specified time window [7]. The computer will then send a reminder to the patient in the form of a text message, a call to the patient's cell phone, or an e-mail message [7].

These devices will not serve to remedy the lack of compliance in a patient who does not intend on taking the medication in the first place [7]. "If the patient is intent on being noncompliant, these devices can be defeated by opening them and then wasting the medication [7]". Additionally, a patient could remove the medication at the designated time and yet give the medication to someone else. This provides a host of dangers, not only for the non-compliant patient missing his/her medication dose but also to the person who ingests medication prescribed for someone else. Example 1, from this chapter, demonstrates how ingesting a "simple" drug, like an antibiotic, could adversely affect a person it was not prescribed for.

Example 1. Trends In Healthcare: E-Health: Medication Adherence Solutions
Scenario: A 35-year-old woman was prescribed tetracycline (an antibiotic) to treat her rosacea (reddening of the her cheeks and nose). The rosacea began to subside after taking only a few pills. In the meantime, her 5-year-old daughter had developed an ear infection.

The woman gave her remaining vial of medication to her 5-year-old daughter, one pill each day. The mother did not take anymore tetracycline. The infant matured normally with the exception of her teeth. The mother's rosacea returned, but was subsequently treated with another prescription of tetracycline.

Discussion: Tetracycline should almost never be given to children as it permanently discolors the teeth of children. Tetracycline can cause permanent yellowing or graying of the teeth to a child under 8 years old [5]. Therefore, tetracycline exposure during any of these periods of calcification can result in permanent staining [6]. Had the woman completed her regimen, she would not have incurred more health care expense by getting two prescriptions. Also, her daughter would not have to live a life of shame with discolored teeth.

Patients that want to adhere to their medication regimen could also use mobile applications (apps). Such applications could provide visual, audible or vibrating reminders [7].

9.1.2 Social Media Use

Social media allows for you to share your medical condition with others. "Patients can share their experiences through discussion forums, chat rooms and instant messaging, or online consultation with a qualified clinician" [11-14].

Some websites offer patients a source of information about a particular condition and allows for these patients to join a chat room that allows them to discuss their experiences with other patients afflicted by the same condition.

"Although there are several benefits to the use of social media for health communication, the information exchanged needs to be monitored for quality and reliability, and the users' confidentiality and privacy need to be maintained." [11].

9.2 Use of More Healthcare Professionals

9.2.1 Medical Extenders

Medical extenders are the healthcare professionals that were mentioned in Chapter 2.2.2, Doctor Selection: Choosing a Medical Professional with the Best Training to Treat Your Condition: Medical Doctor vs. Other Health Care Professionals. Medical extenders are non-MD healthcare professionals that interact directly with patients. They are nurse practitioners, medical assistants, health educators, social workers, and registered dieticians [15]. Different titles such as "mid-level-provider", "physician extender" and "health care provider" have often been used to describe nurse practitioners (NPs) and physician assistants (PAs) [16].

Some say that there will be a shortage of U.S. doctors in the future. There are many possible reasons for this including the rise in power of insurance companies, more people having access to healthcare secondary to healthcare reform, and the litigious nature of the legal system against healthcare professionals. Regardless of the reason, medical extenders will play an ever-increasing role not only in the delivery of care, but also the ongoing nurturing of patient relationships [15]. Medical extenders will be needed in places where doctors are not available, such as in rural settings. "Considerable federal dollars have been allocated to train more NPs and PAs, respectively, over a ten-year period to help reduce the shortages in primary care, the backbone of preventative care" [16]. "NPs and PAs can be educated in a shorter period of time than physicians, thus supplying communities with much-needed primary care health providers in a timely fashion" [16].

9.2.2 The Virtual Doctor: Telemedicine

Telemedicine is the study and practice of medicine in a virtual setting. It uses communications networks for delivery of healthcare services and medical education from one geographical location to another [17].

This means that healthcare professionals can use technology to communicate and "practice" medicine without seeing the patient in person. It is another benefit of e-Health. Telemedicine can become an extremely useful tool for supplying remote areas with "virtual" medical personnel. It can also be used from one office to the next when a doctor is searching for a "second" opinion from a colleague. The colleague could be miles away, even on a different continent and yet could render his/her opinion about a patient.

Telemedicine uses the Internet and/or cellphone services to transmit images of the patient to the doctor. A doctor can see these images on his/her computer or phone. This allows for the doctor to be anywhere in the world and see a patient from anywhere else in the world, as long as there is strong Internet connection and/or cellphone service. Keep in mind, that the doctor is literally "seeing " the patient or a part of the patient, but cannot touch the patient. Therefore, such doctors render a diagnosis but must rely upon local healthcare professionals to treat the patient.

Doctors who practice medicine that do not require touching patients are best served by telemedicine. Such doctors include the "hidden" doctors (radiologists and pathologists) as mentioned in Chapter 2.4, Doctor Selection: The "Hidden" Doctor You "Cannot" Choose. These doctors diagnose a patient's condition but do not physically touch the patient. Depending on the case, a dermatologist may also not need to touch the patient. (For example, a dermatologist can see acne and does not need to touch it to treat it. Instead, the dermatologist can contact the patient's pharmacy to prescribe the acne medication.) Psychiatrists also do not necessarily require touching the patient and could potentially use telecommunication (talking with a patient via a computer screen) to practice telemedicine.

The potential draw back of telemedicine is that opinions can only be rendered on cases that do not require touching the patient. In other words, performing a physical examination or surgery on a patient is not possible using telemedicine because the doctor is not physically in the room with the patient. However, in time, doctors may be able to instruct robots to perform procedures, while the doctors can monitor the robot's progress from a screen, miles away. Although robots and computers can not replace the human bond between a patient and a physician, they could serve to improve healthcare in regions of the world that lack medical professionals, like in remote villages, in the country side or abandoned cities.

As of now, there are few standards and guidelines for doctors to comply with while performing telemedicine [18]. This will change, as issues of safety, patient privacy, medical legal and doctor reimbursement, must be addressed.

9.3   Individualized Medicine: Potential Treatment Options...?

9.3.1 Stem cells

A stem cell is a cell with the capability of becoming a different cell. Stem cells can turn into any type of cell in the body, like heart cells, muscles or neurons [19].

A stem cell develops into any cell type when it is given nutrients. The type of nutrients given determines which type of cell it will grow into. Grown up cells are called differentiated cells. The accumulation of numerous differentiated cells, leads to the development of tissue and organs. Thus, stem cells can potentially form tissues and organs, depending on the type of nutrients they are given.

"Because stem cells can give rise to any tissue found in the body, they provide nearly limitless potential for medical applications" [20]. At this time, stem cells provide life-saving treatments for patients with leukemia, lymphoma, other blood disorders, and some solid tumors [20].

"Current studies are researching how stem cells may be used to prevent or cure diseases and injuries such as Parkinson's disease, type 1 diabetes, heart disease, spinal cord injury, Duchene's muscular dystrophy, Alzheimer's disease, strokes, burns, osteoarthritis, rheumatoid arthritis, vision, and hearing loss. Stem cells could also be used someday to replace or repair tissue damaged by disease or injury" [20].

There are two types of stem cells: embryonic and adult. The type of stem cells that can develop into almost any other type of cell (as in the process described above) is the embryonic stem cell. For this reason, the embryonic stem cell is the preferred cell for scientists to study.

The other type of stem cell is the adult stem cell. It can easily be obtained from skin, hair, and saliva. But the adult stem cell cannot be treated by scientists to become any other cell type without first manipulating it. The manipulation of the adult stem cell involves transforming it into an embryonic stem cell. Thus, the adult stem cell must first be manipulated to become like an embryonic stem cell [19]. It is called a pluripotent stem cell [19]. After this step, like a pure embryonic stem cell, it can then be given nutrients to change into any other type of cell, tissue or organ.

Natural embryonic stem cells are difficult to retrieve and raise regulatory and ethical issues. There are also regulatory and ethical barriers for the use of some stem cells (embryonic stem cells) [20]. This is mostly because of the manner in which these stem cells are retrieved and/or created. "Human embryonic cells are now mainly derived from embryos created by fertilization in fertility clinics" [19].

9.3.2 Cloning

Cloning is replicating the exact genetic makeup of a plant, animal or human. At this time, few researchers are using cloning to obtain embryonic stem cells. (As explained in the previous Section 9.3.1, Stem Cells, scientists prefer using embryonic stem cells as opposed to adult stem cells. But obtaining embryonic stem cells has moral, ethical and legal restrictions.) To obtain embryonic stem cells from cloning, researchers could do the following:

> Remove an adult stem cell from the skin of a patient. Insert the genetic material from the skin cell into a human egg that has been previously stripped of its own genetic material. An embryo should develop (as

the genetic material from the skin represents some of the patient's mother and father's genetic code). Embryonic stem cells can then be retrieved from the newly created embryo. (The potential use of embryonic stem cells is explained in the previous Section 9.3.1, Stem Cells.)

If the embryo is capable of further growth and development by the addition of "growth nutrients", it can become a clone. ("Growth nutrients" have not been well established in the science community and is one of the reasons for the inability to produce viable clones.)

The benefit of human cloning is that the clone's organs could be used to replace the patient's diseased organ. When using a cloned organ, the patient should avoid rejection of the organ, as the cloned organ is genetically the same as the patient's. Cloning would allow for hundreds of patients on transplant waiting lists to receive an organ, namely one derived from himself/herself.

The moral issue surrounding human cloning is obvious. There are fears that people would use this technology for dangerous, self-serving purposes including the creation of armies to serve as soldiers or slaves. "The first human clone will probably be born outside the United States-perhaps in China, where work on human cloning is reported to be proceeding" [21].

9.3.3 Transplant

When a patient has an organ, such as a liver, kidney, heart or lung that is failing, a new one is needed. Scientists are constantly researching new ways to resolve this life threatening issue. A device like a dialysis machine attempts to do some of the function of a failing or missing kidney, for example. However, it does not fully replace the kidney and complications can arise over time. Therefore, scientists continue to develop new forms of therapy for failing organs.

One such development is the use of 3-D printing for organ support, organ transplant and the reconstruction of other body parts. This technology requires a selected material to be printed out from a printer in the shape desired for its use. So, the printer will spew out a product the very shape of a blood vessel, if that is what it has been programmed to create. Ideally, overlying this material are stem cells. The stem cells overlying the printed material will grow and mature into the strong adult cells that should be found in the body tissue/organ it is replacing. Coating the material with stem cells should prevent rejection. The material represents scaffolding that the stem cells are allowed to grow and develop on. Ultimately, you are left with a model of the original tissue/organ.

In 2012, 3-D printing was successfully used by the University of Michigan in the construction of a small device to keep an infant's windpipe open [22]. The infant suffered from a birth defect of his windpipe and had a 3-D splint inserted to offer support to keep his windpipe open [22]. A splint does not replace the existing organ but is used to add support. In this case, the splint was inserted to keep the existing windpipe open and functioning properly [22].

In 2013, at Children's Hospital of Illinois in Peoria, a child with a diseased windpipe had it replaced using 3-D technology with stem cells [24]. In this case, 3-D printed material was printed with overlying layers of stem cells. The stem cells grew and multiplied overtime and conformed to their environment. Using stem cells, which were taken from the patient's own fat or bone marrow, virtually eliminated the patient's body rejecting the transplant [23].

The structural material used in 3-D printing varies depending on the laboratory that is working on it and which type of organ they are trying to recreate. In the case of the University of Michigan, resorbable material was used to construct a splint [22]. Resorbable means that the material used will eventually deteriorate or melt away while inside the patient's body, leaving behind the stem cells that were overlying it. Thus, after the resorbable material has disappeared, all that will remain are the stem cells that should have matured into strong cells, capable of performing their duty, without the underlying presence of the originally scaffolding.

Yet, in the case at Children's Hospital in Peoria, non-absorbable nanofibers were used when constructing a windpipe [24]. Thus, the scaffolding will remain in the patient's body, along with the overlying, matured stem cells. Vitamin B is being tested in one laboratory to reduce some potential toxic effects when using other ingredients when building the printed structure [25].

Sy Mukherjee described the top 5 promising uses of 3-D printing in medicine:

- "Cutting down the backlogged kidney transplant list.
- Regulating diabetes by creating *entirely new* organs.
- Grafting skin onto burn victims
- Making prostheses resemble the original missing limb
- Addressing poor Americans' dental health needs" [26]

Currently, the potential problem with 3-D printing is the structure of the product itself. For example, if attempting to print a complex organ, the 3-D structure may lack the strength and complexities of the original organ [23]. Also, as mentioned above, reducing the possible toxic effects of the material used as scaffolding that underlies the stem cells must be addressed.

9.3.4 Cancer Treatment

Cancer is a change in a normal cell that gives that cell the capability of growing and multiplying beyond that of a normal cell. Thus, because of this capability, the normal cell becomes an abnormal cell, known as cancer. Historically, treatment of cancer involved surgically removing the cancerous growth. This technique is still used today.

Around 1896, radiation therapy was introduced as another form of treatment against cancer [27]. Unfortunately, with radiation therapy, normal cells are also killed because the radiation beam does not specifically target the cancer cells. The destruction of some normal cells is the reason for some of the side effects experienced by patients using radiation therapy.

In the 1940s, chemotherapy was introduced to maximize the effects of surgery or to be used on its own [28]. In general, chemotherapy works by seeking to obliterate cancer cells. Unfortunately, like radiation therapy, both cancer cells and normal cells are affected. Again, the destruction of some normal cells is the reason for some of the side effects experienced by patients on chemotherapy.

Cancer may be effectively treated with the use of surgery, chemotherapy or radiation therapy, or by a combination of all therapies.

In the late 1990s, scientists developed targeted therapies that influence the processes that control growth, division, and spread of cancer cells, as well as the signals that cause cancer cells to die naturally [29]. Thus, fewer normal cells would be affected. Such a practice would reduce side effects, as many normal cells would be allowed to survive and function. Unfortunately, only a few drugs have been successful in this feat. They include drugs that target hormonal sites on cancer cells in some breast cancers, genes in some leukemia and some other cancers. (For a list of targeted cancer therapies, go to http://www.cancer.gov/cancertopics/factsheet/Therapy/targeted.)

- The eventual goal of targeted cancer therapy is to create individualized treatments based on the unique set of molecular targets produced by the patient's own tumor [30]. In other words, different medication would be developed specifically for each patient afflicted with cancer. Ideally, as more targeted cancer therapies are developed, they will be more selective for cancer cells than normal cells, thus harming fewer normal cells, reducing side effects, and improving quality of life [30].

- Targeted therapies have some limitations, such as cancer cells developing resistance to them [30]. For this reason targeted therapies may work best in combination, either with other targeted therapies or with more traditional therapies, such as surgery, chemotherapy and radiation therapy [30].

9.3.5 Gene Therapy

"Genes are the building blocks of inheritance. Passed from parent to child, they contain instructions for making proteins. If genes don't produce the right proteins or don't produce them correctly, a child can have a genetic disorder" [31].

Gene therapy is designed to introduce genetic material into abnormal cells [32]. In most literature, the abnormal cells are called mutated cells. Gene therapy strives to add new genes (proteins) into a mutated cell so that the cell begins to produce normal genes (proteins).

In gene therapy, the new gene (protein) must be carried into the mutated cell. This carrier is called a vector and is genetically engineered to deliver the gene [32]. The vector can be injected or given intravenously (by IV) directly into a specific tissue in the body and is taken up by individual cells [32]. Alternately, a sample of the patient's cells can be removed and exposed to the vector in a laboratory setting [32]. The cells containing the vector are then returned to the patient [32].

"Gene therapy is an experimental technique that uses genes to treat or prevent diseases, including inherited disorders, some types of cancer, and certain viral infections" [32]. "In the future, this technique may allow doctors to treat a disorder by inserting a gene into a patient's cells instead of using drugs or surgery" [32].

"Researchers are testing several approaches to gene therapy, including:

- Replacing a mutated gene that causes disease with a healthy copy of the gene.
- Inactivating, or "knocking out," a mutated gene that is functioning improperly.
- Introducing a new gene into the body to help fight a disease" [32].
- Although gene therapy is a promising treatment option for a number of diseases, researchers must overcome many technical challenges before gene therapy can be

used safely and effectively [32]. For example, scientists must find better ways to deliver new genes and target them to specific mutated cells [32]. Scientists must prevent the production of a dangerous version of a gene (protein) [32]. They must also prevent the overproduction of a good gene (protein), as too much good gene (protein) in a cell can cause the cell to die from toxicity [33].

As of November 2013, gene therapy is only being tested for the treatment of diseases that have no other cures [32].

9.4 Policy Updates

9.4.1 Accountable Care Organizations
In order to reduce the cost of healthcare, a solution was needed to accomplish this. One such potential solution is an Accountable Care Organization (ACO). An ACO is a network of healthcare professionals and institutions that have agreed to take care of a patient, together. An ACO must have one primary care doctor as the "leader" of the patient's overall care. (For more information on primary care doctors, please see Chapter 1.2, Basic Medical Knowledge: Who are Primary Care Doctors?)

Other members of the network could include other physicians, specialists, hospitals and even private pharmacies. "ACOs make providers jointly accountable for the health of their patients, giving them financial incentives to cooperate and save money by avoiding unnecessary tests and procedures" [34].

The goal of ACOs is to deliver healthcare in the most medically and cost efficient manner possible. In order to achieve this, ACOs coordinate care by sharing all electronic medical records, between providers, belonging to a patient. This includes: diagnosis, treatments (physical and medication), tests and billing. This allows for expedient, automatic healthcare updates regarding your medical chart. So, when you travel between appointments, a doctor will have access to your record from the other doctors. (This technology is further explained in this chapter, Section 9.1.1, E-Health: Patient And Administrative Office Benefits.) However, patients belonging to ACOs can see doctors of their choice outside the network without paying more and can decline to have his/her data shared within the ACO [34].

Additionally, ACOs have agreed to be paid via a system that rewards quality outcomes [35]. With this system, doctors and hospitals have to meet specific quality benchmarks, focusing on prevention and carefully managing patients with chronic diseases [34]. The goal is to pay the healthcare professionals more if they keep their patients well and out of the hospital [34].

In order to encourage more doctors to join an ACO, the government offers financial incentives to doctors' offices that join and comply with the ACO guidelines. "ACOs doctors can choose to be at risk of losing money if they want to aim for a bigger reward, or they can enter the program with no risk at all" [34]. Despite these financial incentives, many doctors do not want to join for various reasons, most often due to the cost and time needed to set up the program in their office.

As of Summer 2013, an estimated 14 percent of the U.S. population belonged to an ACO, including approximately four million Medicare beneficiaries [34]. ACOs could save Medicare up to $940 million in the first four years and if successful, it can be expanded by the federal secretary of the

Department of Health and Human Services [34]. In a study done to examine the success of the most engaged ACOs (those belonging to the Pioneers program), the 32 ACOs succeeded in improving quality and performed better than fee-for-service Medicare in 15 quality measures; they generated a gross savings of $87.6 million in 2012, the first year of the program [34].

Bringing your medications to your new appointment was encouraged in Chapter 3.1, Preparation For The First Medical Visit: Planning for the First Medical Visit, however, ACOs have access to this list automatically, so there would be no need to carry them. Thus, you would not need to bring your medications to your new appointment if your doctors are members of an ACO. Ask your doctor's office staff, if your doctor is a member of an ACO. If your doctor is not a member, then he/she will not have access to all of your records from other doctors.

Summary: Trends In Healthcare

- **By opening communication, E-Health offers advantages to patients, doctors, insurance companies and governmental agencies.**
- **You may be seen by an alternate healthcare professional: the medical extender or the virtual doctor.**
- **Individualized (personalized) medicine: Scientists are developing unique advances that are based on each individual patient, to treat devastating diseases and conditions.**
- **The government intends to have fewer uninsured Americans, improve the health of all Americans and decrease the overall cost of healthcare, most notably by focusing on preventative care.**

References

1. World Health Organization. E-Health. <u>Retrieved 2013, November 18, from</u> http://www.who.int/trade/glossary/story021/en/

2. Open Clinical: Knowledge Management for Medical Care. E-Health. Retrieved 2013, November 18, from (http://www.openclinical.org/e-Health.html)

3. Garret, P. and Seidman, J. (2011, January 4). EMR vs EHR- What is the Difference? Health IT Buzz. Retrieved 2013, November 18 from, http://www.healthit.gov/buzz-blog/electronic-health-and-medical-records/emr-vs-ehr-difference/

4. Abha Agrawal. (2009). Medication Errors: Prevention Using Information Technology Systems. *Br J Clin Pharmacol.* June; 67 (6): 681-686.

5. Tetracycline. Drugs.com. Retrieved on 2013, December 18 from http://www.drugs.com/tetracycline.html.

6. Pharmacology Weekly. March 16, 2009. Part 1: How Does the Antibiotic Tetracycline Cause Permanent Staining of the Teeth and Who is at Risk? Retrieved 2013, December 15 from, http://www.pharmacologyweekly.com/custom/archived-content/drug-interactions/39.

7. Figge, HL. Electronic Tools to Measure and Enhance Medication Adherence. *Allscripts Chicago, Illinois.* 4/20/2011. *US Pharm.* 2010;36(4) (Compliance & Adherence suppl):6-10. Retrieved 2013, December 12 from http://www.uspharmacist.com/content/s/162/c/27847/12/12/13.

8. Koehler AM, and Maibach HI. (2001). Electronic Monitoring in Medication Adherence Measurement. Implications for Dermatology. *Am J Clin Dermatol.* 2(1):7-12.

9. Wantland DJ, Portillo CJ, Holzemer WL, Slaughter R, McGhee EM. The Effectiveness of Web-based vs. Non-Web-Based Interventions: A Meta-analysis of Behavioral Change Outcomes. J Med Internet Res. 2004 Nov 10;6(4):e40. Retrieved from http://www.jmir.org/2004/4/e40/v6e40. doi: 10.2196/jmir.6.4.e40.

10. Nieuwkerk, P and Carl Stepnowsky C (Reviewers). Effects of eHealth Interventions on Medication Adherence: A Systematic Review of the Literature. Eysenbach, G (Ed).(2011). *Med Internet Res.* 2011 Oct-Dec; 13(4): e103. doi: 10.2196/jmir.1738.

11. Moorhead SA, Hazlett DE, Harrison L, Carroll JK, Irwin A, and Hoving C. A New Dimension of Health Care: Systematic Review of the Uses, Benefits, and Limitations of Social Media for Health Communication. *J Med Internet Res.* 2013 Apr 23;15(4):e85. doi: 10.2196/jmir.1933.

12. Adams SA. Blog-based Applications and Health Information: Two Case Studies that Illustrate Important Questions for Consumer Health Informatics (CHI) research. *Int J Med Inform.* 2010 Jun;79(6):e89–96. doi: 10.1016/j.ijmedinf.2008.06.009.

13. Hwang KO, Ottenbacher AJ, Green AP, Cannon-Diehl MR, Richardson O, Bernstam EV, and Thomas EJ. Social Support in an Internet Weight Loss Community. *Int J Med Inform.* 2010 Jan;79(1):5–13. doi: 10.1016/j.ijmedinf.2009.10.003. Retrieved from http://europepmc.org/abstract/MED/19945338.

14. Kim K, Kwon N. Profile of e-patients: Analysis of Their Cancer Information-Seeking From a National Survey. *J Health Commun.* 2010 Oct;15(7):712–33. doi: 10.1080/10810730.2010.514031.)

15. Healthcare Technology Online. (2013, February 8). Retrieved 2013, November 18 from http://www.healthcaretechnologyonline.com/doc/technology-the-rise-of-the-healthcare-extender-0001.

16. Smith, Darron and Sabino, T. <u>Where's the Doctor? PAs and NPs on the Front Lines of U.S. Healthcare.</u> Retrieved 2013, November 18 from, http://www.academia.edu/1212332/Wheres_the_Doctor_PAs_and_NPs_on_the_Front_Lines_of_U.S._Healthcare.

17. Sood S, Mbarika V, Jugoo S, Dookhy R, Doarn CR, Prakash N, and Merrell RC. What is Telemedicine? A Collection of 104 Peer-Reviewed Perspectives and Theoretical Underpinnings. *Telemed J E Health.* 2007 Oct;13(5):573-90.

18. Krupinski EA, Antoniotti N, and Bernard J. Utilization of the American Telemedicine Association's Clinical Practice Guidelines. *Telemed J E Health.* 2013 Nov;19(11):846-51. doi: 10.1089/tmj.2013.0027.

19. Pollak, A. Cloning Is Used to Create Embryonic Stem Cells. (May 15, 2013). NYTimes. Science. Retrieved 2013, November 30 from http://www.nytimes.com/2013/05/16/science/scientists-use-cloning-to-create-embryonic-stem-cells.html?_r=1&.

20. Basics of Stem Cell Research. American Medical Association. Retrieved 2013, November 30 from http://www.ama-assn.org//ama/pub/physician-resources/medical-science/.

21. Kevles, DJ. Cloning Can't Be Stopped. Wherever the Technology is Satisfactorily Created, Who Will Monitor and Control Its Uses…? (2002, June 1). MIT Technology Review. Retrieved 2013, December 1 from http://

www.technologyreview.com/featuredstory/401460/
cloning-cant-be-stopped/page/2/.

22. Bioresorbable Airway Splint Created with a Three-
Dimensional Printer. (2013, May 23). N Engl J Med
2013; 368:2043-2045. Retrieved 2013, November 30 from
http://www.nejm.org/doi/full/10.1056/NEJMc1206319.
DOI: 10.1056/NEJMc1206319.

23. Huang, J. 3D Printing Organs. (2013, October 16). *In
Applied Sciences, Biological Sciences. Dartmouth.edu. Retrieved
2013. November 29 from http://dujs.dartmouth.edu/biological_
sciences/6026#.UpgWd5X3Bpk.*

24. World's First Trachea Transplant Performed at
Children's Hospital of Illinois. (2013, April 30). OSF
Healthcare. *Retrieved 2013, November 30* from http://www.
osfhealthcare.org/news/2013/release-04302013-001.html.

25. Singh, M. Why Engineers Want To Put B
Vitamins In 3-D Printers.(2013, October 25).
Retrieved 2013, December 11 from http://www.
npr.org/blogs/health/2013/10/24/240566819/
why-engineers-want-to-put-b-vitamins-in-3-d-printers.

26. Mukherjee, S. The 5 Most Promising Uses
of 3-D Printing in Medicine. Thinkprogress.
org Retrieved 2013, November 28 from, http://
thinkprogress.org/health/2013/05/23/2054281/
promising-uses-3d-printing-medicine/).

27. Tools for Healing. Pulse Accelerator Science in
Medicine. Retrieved 2013, December 11 from, http://
www.fnal.gov/pub/pulse/healing_1.html.

28. History of Chemotherapy. (2010, January 7)
StudentScholarships.org. Retrieved 2013, December 11
from http://www.articlesbase.com/technology-articles/

history-of-chemotherapy-studentscholarshipsorg-1682274.
html.

29. Evolution of Cancer Treatments: Targeted Therapy.
(2012, June 8). The American Cancer Society.
Retrieved 2013, December 11 from, http://www.
cancer.org/cancer/cancerbasics/thehistoryofcancer/
the-history-of-cancer-cancer-treatment-targeted-therapy

30. Targeted Cancer Therapy. (2012, December 5).
National Cancer Institute at the National Institutes of
Health. Retrieved 2013, December 1 from, http://www.
cancer.gov/cancertopics/factsheet/Therapy/targeted on
12/1/13.

31. A Service of the U.S. National Library of Medicine.
Medline Plus: Trusted Health Information for You.
National Institutes of Health. Retrieved 2013, December
1 from, http://www.nlm.nih.gov/medlineplus/
genesandgenetherapy.html.

32. What is Gene Therapy? (2013, November 25). National
Institute of Health. Retrieved December 1, 2013,
December 1 from http://ghr.nlm.nih.gov/handbook/
therapy/genetherapy.

33. Young, S. New Genome-Editing Method Could Make
Gene Therapy More Precise and Effective. (November
27, 2013). MIT Technology Review. Retrieved 2013,
December 1, from http://www.technologyreview.com/
news/522051/new-genome-editing-method-could-make-
gene-therapy-more-precise-and-effective/

34. Gold, J. FAQ On ACOs: Accountable Care
Organizations, Explained. ACO is the Hottest Three-
Letter Word in Health Care. Kaiser Health News. 2013,
Aug 23). Retrieved on 2013, December 3, from http://

www.kaiserhealthnews.org/stories/2011/january/13/aco-accountable-care-organization-faq.aspx

35. Why is Health Care Delivery Reform as Proposed in the Affordable Care Act Necessary?. Accountable Care Facts. Retrieved 2013, December 3 from http://www.accountablecarefacts.org/topten/what-are-the-barriers-and-challenges-such-organizations-might-face-1

Afterword

ARMED WITH THE INFORMATION IN THIS book, a patient should be able to navigate through the healthcare system with confidence. The patient equipped with this information is better prepared to tackle and prevent potential healthcare related problems.

Ignorance can lead to victimization. Knowledge, on the other hand, can result in respect and better treatment. The same is true in medicine. If you come to a medical visit prepared, you can expect better service from the entire office staff. This book prepares its readers with the basic knowledge needed to accomplish this.

As reviewed in this book, patients need to understand; the basics of medicine, the difference between medical specialties, the importance of their medical office visit, the need for medical insurance and disability insurance, identifying medical fraud and malpractice and finally, knowing about current trends in medical technology. This book offers this information in great detail and serves as a comprehensive "self-help" book for patients. If you are aware of your "rights" within the healthcare system, you are better equipped to prevail!